The Beginner's Ketogenic Diet for Health Benefits and Weight Loss

Includes a 30 Day Meal Plan with 100 Keto Diet Recipes, and a Sample Shopping List

Introduction 10

Chapter One: Overview of Keto Diet.......................13
What is It? 13
How it Works? 13
Who Can Follow the Keto Diet? 14
What Can I Eat While Following This Diet? 15
Fruit...15
Vegetables 15
Protein & Fats 16
What Not to Eat? 16
Starch & Carbs 16
Sugar 17
Alcohol...17

Chapter Two: Benefits and Risks of the Keto Diet 18
Regulates Your Appetite...18
Helps in Managing Your Blood Sugar Levels 19
Helps in Regulating Your Blood Pressure Levels 20
Get Rid of Visceral Fat..21
Helps in Reducing Triglyceride Levels 22
Increases the High-Density Lipoprotein (HDL)
Cholesterol Levels...23
Increases Low Density Lipoprotein (LDL) Cholesterol
Patterns 23
Prescribed for Patients Suffering from Cognitive
Disorders...24
Helps in Losing Weight 24
Helps with Metabolic Syndrome 25
Risks to Consider 26

Chapter Three: Tips to Get Started 28
Start with Your Pantry...28
Go Shopping 29
Read the Labels Before Buying 34
Buy in Bulk Quantities 35
Saves Money 36

Saves Time..36

A Big Source of Motivation 36

Stop Eating Out Before You Begin the Diet..................37

Keep a Tab on the Protein Content............................38

Consume Root Vegetables in Minimal Quantities 39

Formulate Your Own Support Group............................39

No More Peer Pressure 40

Constant Motivation 40

Incorporating Changes 41

Join Social Groups..42

Maintain a Food Journal 44

Managing Social Outings....................................45

Eat Before You Go Out 46

Refuse the Menu Card 46

Let Your Host Know Your Preference.............46

Keep Your Body Hydrated....................................47

Consume Chicken Broth 47

Come Up with a Suitable Reward System 47

Set Tangible Goals First 48

Come Up with Appropriate Rewards..............48

Time Your Rewards Properly.........................49

Rewards Should be in Line with the Diet 49

Be Consistent..50

Track Your Progress 50

Don't Exercise During the First Two Weeks 52

Cook Your Own Meals..52

Be Patient and Learn to Move On 53

Chapter Four: Ketogenic Condiment Recipes 55

Zero Carb Mayonnaise 55

5 Minute Keto Pesto 56

Caesar Dressing 57

Chia Seed and Strawberry Jam 58

Guacamole..59

Chive Egg Dip 60

Egg Fast Alfredo Sauce 61

Chapter Five: Ketogenic Breakfast Recipes............62

3

Cheese and Ham Waffles 62

Bacon, Cheese and Egg Cups 64

Apple and Brie Crepes 66

Zucchini and Chicken Quiche 68

Lemon Poppy Seed Pancakes 72

Feta & Pesto Omelet 73

Perfect Scramble 75

Blackberry Egg Bake 76

Creamy Cauliflower and Ground Beef Skillet 77

Morning Meatloaf 79

Breakfast BLT Salad 81

Chocolate Waffles 82

Liver, Sausage and Eggs...83

Coconut Flour Porridge Breakfast Cereal 84

Chapter Six: Ketogenic Soup Recipes 85

Chicken Kale Soup 85

Avgolemono (Greek Chicken Lemon and Egg Soup) 86

Creamy Garlic Chicken Soup......................................87

Cream of Chicken Soup with Bacon 88

Queso Soup...90

Kale and Sausage Soup...91

Jalapeño Popper Soup 93

Creamy Mushroom, Fennel and Leek Soup.................94

Broccoli Cheese Soup..96

Roasted Red Bell Pepper and Cauliflower Soup 97

Creamy Red Gazpacho 99

Chapter Seven: Ketogenic Smoothie Recipes..........101

Strawberry & Rhubarb Pie Smoothie 101

Fat Bomb Chocolate Smoothie 102

Healthy Keto Green Smoothie 103

Healthy Green Shake 104

Green Lemon Smoothie..105

Strawberry Almond Smoothie....................................106

Coco-Nut Milkshake 107

Orange Creamsicle Cooler..108

Raspberry Avocado Smoothie 109

Blackberry Cheesecake Smoothie 110
Low Carb Smoothie Bowl 111

Chapter Eight: Ketogenic Salad Recipes 112
Crunchy and Nutty Cauliflower Salad 112
Mediterranean Chopped Salad 113
Mock Potato Salad 114
Chicken Salad Picnic Eggs...................................116
Chicken Cobb Salad 118
Lemon Blueberry Chicken Salad..............................119
Curried Chicken Salad 120
Easy Russian Slaw 122
Grilled Vegetable Salad with Olive oil and Feta..........123

Chapter Nine: Ketogenic Snack Recipes.............124
Rainbow Goat's Cheese Balls................................124
Italian Style Zucchini Rolls.................................125
Bacon-Goat Cheese Jalapeno Poppers.......................126
Marinated Olives and Feta 127
Fish Fingers 128
Low Carb Pizza Bites 129
Spicy Chicken Nuggets 130
Mini Cheese Balls...131
Smoked Paprika Zucchini Chips 132
Zucchini Pizza Bites 133
Cucumber Bites 135
Pesto Keto Crackers 138

Chapter Ten: Ketogenic Side Dish Recipes............140
Cauliflower Cheese & Onion Croquettes....................140
Cheese and Jalapeño Bread.................................142
Cheesy Cauliflower Gratin...................................144
Colcannon 145
Loaded Mashed Cheesy Pancetta Cauliflower...........146
Coconut Tortillas 148
Creamy Greek Zucchini Patties 149
2-Minute Low Carb English Muffins.........................151
Creamy Ricotta Spaghetti Squash 153
Spicy Sriracha Roasted Broccoli............................154

Cheesy Asparagus 155
Pork Rind Tortillas 156
Almond Flour Cream Cheese Crepes.....................157

Chapter Eleven: Ketogenic Main Course Recipes ...158
Broccoli Chicken Zucchini Boats 158
Sesame Ginger Chicken..160
Baked Mediterranean Chicken 161
Bacon, Avocado, and Chicken Sandwich.................163
Zucchini Pizza Casserole 165
Spinach and Feta Turkey Burgers 167
Mediterranean Pork Chops 168
Broccoli Rabe & Italian Sausage 170
Southwestern Pork Stew 171
Cheese Pizza Rolls 173
Low Carb Beef Burritos 175
Mexican Shredded Beef 176
Steak with Mushroom Port Sauce...........................178
Italian Casserole 180
Easy 30 Minute Keto Chili 182
Easy Pan Seared Lamb Chops with Mustard Cream
Sauce 184
Spicy Tuna Poke Bowl 186
Walnut Crusted Salmon 188
Thai Shrimp Curry 189
Spicy Shrimp and Cabbage Stir Fry.........................191
Mediterranean Cauliflower Pizza 193
Tempeh Lettuce Wraps...195
Egg Florentine 197
Grain Free Mac and Cheese 198

Chapter Twelve: Ketogenic Dessert Recipes...........199
Maple Pecan Muffins 203
Coconut Mocha Mug Cake.......................................206
Blackberry Pudding 207
Strawberry Shortcake...209
Dreamsicle Dessert 211
Chocolate Ice Cream..212

Frost Bite Cookies 213

Chapter Thirteen: 30-day Meal Plan.......................215

Conclusion 224

Recommended Reading..225

Recommended Websites (under development) 226

Recommended Products and Solutions (Future) ...227

The information herein is offered for informational purposes solely, and is universal as so. The presentation of the information is without contract or any type of guarantee assurance.

DISCLAIMER: *Everyone, regardless of their condition, should first consult with their physician or medical professional and receive formal medical clearance before starting any diet, lifestyle change or exercise program.*

This publisher and author are not licensed or medical practitioners and do not provide any medical advice whatsoever. The publisher and author claim no responsibility to anyone or entity for any liability, loss, or damage caused or allegedly caused by use of the information presented in this publication.

The trademarks that are used are without any consent, and the publication of the trademark is without permission or backing by the trademark owner. All trademarks and brands within this book are for clarifying purposes only and are the owned by the owners themselves, not affiliated with this document.

Introduction

I want to thank you and congratulate you for purchasing the book, *"The Beginner's Ketogenic Diet for Health Benefits and Weight Loss."*

Trying to stay healthy is almost regarded as a chore these days. Gone are the days when we didn't have to worry about what we eat, because we were familiar with the ingredients that went into the dish. With globalization, there are so many options available today.

We often go by the taste and choose our dishes without really understanding how well our bodies will accept a different cuisine or the nutritional content of these dishes. If that is not scary enough, we don't really know how the things that we add to our shopping cart so easily, are processes and actually laden with artificial preservatives and ingredients. With the surge of junk foods, staying healthy is a separate project all by itself.

The alarming increase in the number of people suffering from chronic and lifestyle disorders is definitely serving as an eye opener and making us reevaluate our choices. Being unhealthy and obese are not something that anybody can overlook, considering the negative risk factors associated with obesity.

Trying to lose weight will only solve one part of the problem. Unfortunately, many fail to realize that. I learned this the hard way.

People end up trying one diet plan after another, with the intention of just losing weight and don't really understand the reason behind the risk factors for several lifestyle related disorders.

When each diet plan doesn't really improve the quality of their lifestyle, they only end up getting frustrated! Sound familiar? I faced the exact same issue.

Well, it's time to end your chase behind such one-dimensional diet plans. It's time you switched to a diet which is **holistic in its approach towards improving the quality of your life**.

Say hello to the ketogenic diet! This diet is not just **designed for weight loss but more importantly for improved health benefits as well**. The benefits of this diet are several and you will be amazed with how this singular diet is capable of addressing various risk factors at once.

If this is the first time you have come across the ketogenic diet, don't worry. You have done the right thing by choosing this book. This book contains relevant information that you need to know, before you implement **this lifestyle** diet.

The **first chapter** of this book **will give you a brief overview of what this diet is** all about. This chapter will help you to get an understanding on the principles of this diet.

The **second chapter highlights the various benefits** of following this diet. The **third chapter** contains several **useful tips**, which will help you implement this diet and follow it religiously, without succumbing to deviations.

To motivate you, I have also provided a **30 day Keto Diet meal plan, more than 100 Keto Diet friendly recipes, and a sample shopping list** as part of the later chapters.

I am sure that you will be glad that you came across this diet plan! From my personal experience, I would say that this is much more than just a diet plan. **It is a welcome lifestyle change!** I hope you find this book useful.

Thanks again for purchasing this book. I hope you enjoy it!

Chapter One: Overview of Keto Diet

We will first take a look at the basics of the Keto diet in this section of the book. We will also go over some of the basic questions and concepts, like what exactly is the Keto diet, the key factors that differentiate it from some other health focused diets, the basic science behind how the diet works, the feasibility of the diet for people with other health issues and finally, and most importantly, what you can and cannot eat as part of the diet. Let's get started!

What is It?

Dealing with the most basic question first, the Keto Diet is a specific form of diet that aims to create a certain kind of calorie deficit situation in the body, that will drive the body into a state called ***Ketosis*** (now you know where the name for the diet came from!). During Ketosis, the liver looks for the energy stored in the body in the form of fat and produce ketones. I will get into the mechanics of it in a bit!

As part of the Keto Diet, you will need to cut down on the amount of carbohydrates consumed and focus more on fats. ***This is a high fat and low carb diet*** but don't be alarmed until you read further about the Keto Diet. This diet also encourages you to consume adequate protein!

How it Works?

Let's see how this diet works now! As part of the digestive process, our body breaks down the carbohydrates present in the food into glucose. This is done by our digestive system because glucose is the quickest and easiest route for generating energy. As I mentioned earlier, this diet is all about decreasing your consumption of carbs. By following the Keto

Diet, *you are actually attempting to reduce the production of glucose, thereby making the body to go into the ketosis state, where it taps into the stored fats*.

But making the body go into a complete calorie-deficit state may not always be the right thing to do. This is why simply starving will not help you achieve ketosis. The *Keto Diet is not about depriving your body of food*. It's more about depriving it of glucose so that it would resort to burning fats for energy.

When the body taps into the fat stored, as a result of ketosis, the process results in the synthesis of ketones. And this ultimately results in your energy needs being met. Production of ketones in this manner has more benefits than meet the eye. In addition to the obvious benefit of providing energy, your basic metabolism rate also increases. You will see shortly how improved metabolism aids in losing weight.

Who Can Follow the Keto Diet?

Before the recent boom in the whole "fitness scene," the Keto Diet used to be prescribed by dieticians for epilepsy patients. Many studies and real-world cases have shown how this diet has worked really well for such patients by complementing their specific medication much better than a normal high-carb diet.

Over the years, this diet is being followed by people to improve the quality of their lifestyles. In fact, this is one of the most effective diets to adopt, if the primary objectives are to lose weight and become healthier, without resorting to any drastic lifestyle changes.

Therefore, it is quite clear that the keto diet can be followed by anyone, provided certain basic precautions are observed. For instance, pregnant women and people over the age of 75 should not consider following this diet. Similarly, people recovering from any major surgery should not be considering the keto diet.

DISCLAIMER: *Everyone, regardless of their condition, should first consult with their physician or medical professional and receive formal medical clearance before starting any diet, lifestyle change or exercise program.*

This publisher and author are not licensed or medical practitioners and do not provide any medical advice whatsoever. The publisher and author claim no responsibility to anyone or entity for any liability, loss, or damage caused or allegedly caused by use of the information presented in this publication.

What Can I Eat While Following This Diet?

Given below are the broad categories of foods that you should be eating more, as part of the Keto diet.

Fruit

Sufficient consumption of fruit has multiple benefits here. On one hand, it is an irreplaceable source of essential fiber in your diet. On the other hand, sweet fruits serve as a healthy replacement of sugar in your diet and can be used as dessert after a meal, in the place of other conventional food items loaded with processed sugar.

Also, fresh fruit is a great source of other minerals and nutrients that you seldom find in other food sources. One caveat is to stay away from high sugar fruits. After all, sugar is sugar no matter the source.

Vegetables

Eating plenty of green leafy vegetables as part of your diet has undeniably great benefits. Just make sure to pick vegetables that are low in carbohydrates (low-glycemic carbs) instead of our usual staples like potatoes and other tubers that are high in carbs.

It is advisable to consume vegetables such as spinach, broccoli, kale, cabbage, cauliflower etc. Vegetables are also loaded with fiber, which can help in regulating your appetite and improving your metabolism.

Protein & Fats

Eating plenty of meat and dairy products, which are rich in fat, is the basic principle behind the Keto diet. Also, remember to consume adequate protein and don't over consume protein which I have seen many do.

Your body needs the protein to repair and heal! You can include chicken and other fowl, beef, mutton, shellfish, fish, cheese, tofu and other unsweetened milk products in your diet. Also make sure the cooking is done in olive oil and butter to support your diet with sufficient amounts of healthy fat.

What Not to Eat?

You should be skipping on the following categories of food, when you are trying to implement this diet:

Starch & Carbs

Avoid starch and excess intake of carbohydrates as much as you can. This means that you will have to get rid of most of your staple dishes, such as porridge, pasta, rice, mashed potatoes and bread. I know this can be quite difficult to implement in the beginning.

I love carbs so this was the hardest for me to avoid. However, you will soon realize that the benefits of keeping them off your plate are several and that should motivate you to avoid them.

Sugar

It goes without saying here that elimination of sugar rich food items is a must when you are following the Keto Diet or any diet. Sugar causes inflammation in your body. Excessively sweet desserts should be avoided at all costs.

You can maybe sneak in a piece of homemade cake or dessert every now and then to satisfy that sweet tooth until you adopt this diet completely! This is extremely hard for many to do but I understand it having been there.

Alcohol

Consuming a glass of wine or whiskey occasionally won't do much harm, but make sure that you stay away from beer. Beer is extremely rich in carbs and you should definitely keep that out of the way!

Did you know that hard liquor such as whiskey, vodka, etc. have no carbs as long as you don't include sweet mixers in the alcohol? This doesn't mean you should drink hard liquor excessively. A drink here or there is fine. I love my single malt scotch!

Chapter Two: Benefits and Risks of the Keto Diet

In this chapter, let's take a look at the several benefits of this diet. Believe me, weight loss is not the only benefit of this diet. You will see shortly how this singular diet is capable of addressing several risk factors at once. This chapter will only leave you with more reassurance that you have done the right thing by choosing this diet.

Regulates Your Appetite

Most often, the reason why I have ended up giving up on a diet plan is because I would feel so tired and hungry. Most diets that I have attempted to follow in the past were so restrictive that I hardly had the satisfaction of eating enough.

The hunger pains and cravings only took a few days to weaken my resolve and I was back on track to eating the way I used to. Sound familiar? I think this applies to most of us.

One of the wonderful things about this diet is that it doesn't make you feel famished except beyond the first few days when your body is still getting used to fat as the source of its energy. When your body starts burning the fat stored, you will feel energized and the high fat content makes you feel full.

It doesn't feel like you are actually dieting because you still get to eat most of the things that you love, except maybe your carbs. *Unlike carbs, fat doesn't get digested quickly*.

Therefore, you won't feel hungry so often. When you consume more carbs, your body burns them off quickly and you end up feeling hungry soon enough. By implementing this diet, you are actually taking care of these random hunger pains and regulating your appetite.

Regulating your appetite also plays an important role in helping you lose weight. When you don't feel hungry often, you will end up eating less than before. Therefore, you only have to worry about an increased number of calories to burn.

Helps in Managing Your Blood Sugar Levels

We have already seen how the intake of carbs is responsible for the release of glucose into our bloodstream. This is the reason why we immediately experience a surge in our energy levels, when we consume carbs.

As you know, the hormone called insulin is responsible for regulating our blood sugar levels. However, insulin doesn't function as it is supposed to, for certain people. It doesn't regulate the blood sugar levels, which results in Type 2 diabetes. This phenomenon of insulin not functioning properly is known as insulin resistance. Therefore, if you are insulin resistant, this diet can help you alleviate the risk of type 2 diabetes. This is because the amount of sugar released into your bloodstream is reduced, as a result of reduced intake of carbs. This way, even if your insulin doesn't function the way it is intended to, your blood sugar levels won't increase and you don't have to worry about type 2 diabetes.

This diet is suitable even if you are suffering from Type 2 diabetes. This diet can actually help you manage your diabetes, with minimal medication, thanks to the reduced production of sugar/glucose.

Helps in Regulating Your Blood Pressure Levels

Hypertension has become a common household problem these days. This is responsible for increasing your risk factors of various disorders related to the kidneys, cardiac disorders etc. Therefore, you simply cannot afford to turn a blind eye to hypertension.

One of the common suggestions prescribed by physicians, as part of treating hypertension, is to reduce your intake of salt. This is because salt is capable of increasing your blood pressure levels.

Well, not all of us can take this suggestion with a pinch of salt, can we? Your meals wouldn't taste the same, without adding salt to them.

Here is the good news – you don't have to cut back on your salt intake, if you are following this diet.

The Keto Diet helps in managing your blood pressure levels, even without reducing your intake of salt. Let's look at how this diet is capable of doing this:

- When you are consuming foods which are rich in carbs, your blood sugar levels will automatically increase. When there is a surge in your blood sugar levels and if you are insulin resistant, it ends up constricting your blood vessels. The constriction in the blood vessels has an impact on your blood pressure levels and causes it to increase.
- By reducing your carb intake, you are essentially managing your blood sugar levels. When your blood sugar is under control, you don't have to worry about constricted blood vessels or hypertension.

- An important reason behind hypertension is insulin resistance. We just saw how the Keto Diet plays an important role in managing your insulin resistance by making you reduce your intake of carbs.
- You will see in a bit how the Keto Diet helps in reducing the amount of visceral fat stored in our bodies. The reduction in the amount of visceral fat helps in managing your insulin resistance. This also helps in lowering your risk factors of several cardiac disorders. With insulin resistance managed, you are reducing one more risk factor for hypertension.
- You already know that this diet encourages the body to burn the fat stored in your body. As part of burning the fat, the sodium and potassium content in your kidneys get flushed out.
- This results in an electrolyte imbalance, which can be addressed by the increased intake of salt and chicken broth. As you can see, you are actually managing your hypertension, with this diet, without reducing your intake of salt.

Get Rid of Visceral Fat

When our body digests the foods that we consume, the fat present gets deposited in different parts of the body which we have no control over where it goes. Depending on the places where our fat gets deposited, the associated risk factors will vary. The fat that we consume gets stored under our skin *(subcutaneous fat)* or gets deposited in the abdominal cavity *(visceral fat)*.

Of these two, *visceral fat is the one that you have to watch out for*. It is extremely dangerous and impacts the quality of your life. It is also capable of affecting the manner in which the different organs in your body function.

When there is an increase in the amount of visceral fat deposited in your body, it causes inflammation of organs, insulin resistance and also impairs your body's metabolism. When the metabolism of your body is impacted, your efforts to lose weight will also be impacted. In fact, it would take you longer than usual to lose weight. Therefore, you have to make sure that your visceral fat deposits are under control.

The Keto Diet is capable of reducing the visceral fat stored in our bodies. This stubborn fat is digested by the body to derive energy. By getting rid of excess visceral fat, you are actually reducing your risk factors for various health disorders. Your efforts to lose weight will also not be compromised by the presence of visceral fat.

Helps in Reducing Triglyceride Levels

When the amount of triglycerides present in your bloodstream increases, it automatically increases your risk of various cardiac disorders. When you consume more carbohydrates, your triglyceride levels will automatically increase.

As you already know, carbs get digested and glucose is released into the bloodstream for energy. If there is excess glucose in the bloodstream, even after your body has derived energy, the insulin secreted by the pancreas converts this excess glucose into triglycerides. These triglycerides are then transported to the fat cells.

When you are not eating, your body derives energy from the release of these stored triglycerides. To put it in simpler terms, increased consumption of carbs paves way to increased levels of triglycerides.

As part of the Keto Diet, you are encouraged to lower or eliminate carbs from your diet. When your carb intake is reduced, you don't have to worry about the presence of excess glucose in your bloodstream or about it getting converted into triglycerides. When the triglyceride levels are regulated, you are taking care of a number of risk factors for several cardiac disorders.

Increases the High-Density Lipoprotein (HDL) Cholesterol Levels

HDL cholesterol is also *known as good cholesterol* and is responsible for ensuring that the cholesterol, present in the food we consume, is transferred to the liver. When the cholesterol reaches the liver, it is either reused by the body for deriving energy or pushed out of the body.

Thus, HDL cholesterol plays an important role in ensuring that the cholesterol content in our food does not end up clogging our arteries. Certain studies also indicate that HDL cholesterol is capable of reducing inflammation. Studies indicate that the Keto Diet is instrumental in improving the levels of HDL cholesterol in our body. This can be attributed to the increased consumption of healthy fats and reduction in the intake of carbs.

Increases Low Density Lipoprotein (LDL) Cholesterol Patterns

LDL cholesterol is also *known as bad cholesterol* and is capable of increasing your risk factors for various cardiac disorders. There is a common misconception that increases in the levels of LDL cholesterol is capable of increasing your risk factors for cardiac disorders.

However, that is not the case. It all comes down to the size of these particles, which determines the impact. Studies indicate that the smaller the particles, greater are the risks for various cardiac disorders. People with larger LDL cholesterol particles suffer from minimal risk of getting cardiac disorders.

Therefore, the size of these particles plays an important role in determining the quality of your lifestyle.

How does the Keto Diet help in increasing the size of these particles?

The sizes of the particles are actually determined by the amount of carbs that you consume. The more carbs you consume, the smaller these particles become. As they get smaller and smaller, the risk factors for cardiac disorders keep increasing by the day. When you follow the Keto Diet, you are actually taking care of your carb intake. Therefore, by reducing your carbs, you are helping in increasing the size of these particles.

Prescribed for Patients Suffering from Cognitive Disorders

We have already seen that this diet is suggested for people, who suffer from epilepsy. This diet complements the medicines prescribed for epilepsy and helps in keeping seizures at bay. This diet is particularly recommended for children, who suffer from epilepsy and don't really respond well to medicines. This diet is also being increasingly prescribed for people, who suffer from cognitive disorders, such as Alzheimer's, Parkinson's etc.

Helps in Losing Weight

This diet definitely helps in accelerating your weight loss. Here is how this diet is effective in helping you lose weight quickly:

- We have already seen how the Keto Diet helps in regulating your appetite. The number of meals that you consume every day would decrease, thanks to the reduced intake of carbs and increased intake of fats. This also helps in accelerating your weight loss.

- When you consume carbs in minimal quantities, the amount of glucose produced is reduced. As a result, the amount of insulin secreted by the body is also reduced. The sodium stored in your kidneys gets flushed out, which helps in reducing your weight.
- Any excess water stored in your body also gets flushed out of the body, as a result of following this diet.
- It is also said that when you consistently follow this diet, expect to lose more weight initially, followed by steady weight loss.

Helps with Metabolic Syndrome

Metabolic syndrome is a disorder, which is an offshoot of the risk factors relating to diabetes and cardiac disorders. Some of the key symptoms associated with the metabolic syndrome are as follows:

- **Abdominal Obesity** – this can be attributed to the high amount of visceral fat stored in the abdominal cavity.
- **Increase in the Blood Sugar Levels** – this can be attributed to the increased intake of carbs.
- **Low HDL Levels** – this could be attributed to the decreased intake of healthy fats.
- **High Blood Pressure Levels** – this can be attributed to obesity, insulin resistance (which is an offshoot of increased intake of carbs)
- **High Triglyceride Levels** – this can be attributed to the increased intake of carbs.

As we have already seen, the Keto Diet is very effective in dealing with the aforesaid symptoms and helping you deal with metabolic syndrome.

These are the several benefits associated with this diet. Weight loss is just one of the many benefits. Don't look at the Keto Diet as a temporary change to your dietary habits.

Incorporate it as part of your lifestyle and lead a healthy life. I cannot think of another diet plan, which is capable of tackling several risk factors at once and contribute so much towards improving the quality of your health. It is indeed a comprehensive diet plan, which can serve as a one-stop solution for various health disorders.

Risks to Consider

While there are numerous benefits to adopting the Keto Diet (really the Keto Lifestyle), I would be remiss if I didn't make you aware of some of the risks. As with any lifestyle and diet change, you need to be fully informed to make the best decision for yourself.

If you don't feel well or think that something isn't right, please immediately see your medical doctor. Don't take any chances.

Some temporary health changes that may occur when you adopt the Keto Diet include the following although this list is not meant to be comprehensive:

- Bad Breath

- Constipation

- Headaches

- Muscle Cramps

- Fatigue

- Nausea

Because excess water will be flushed out of your body, be aware that there could be some mineral and electrolyte deficiencies. At a minimum, you should consider taking a good multi-vitamin with minerals which I what I do. I also recommend that you eat a sufficient amount of green vegetables high in potassium, avocados, low sugar fruit such as berries and nuts.

Chapter Three: Tips to Get Started

Now that you have a basic understanding about this diet and its merits, let's get started.

In this chapter, I have compiled several tips, which will help you get started with this diet and follow it. While this diet is relatively easier to follow, you might still face difficulties initially, while changing your dietary habits.

Patience and perseverance will have to be your best friends, when it comes to implementing any changes to your dietary habits. Therefore, I suggest you follow these tips and be patient with yourself, as you go about implementing this diet.

Start with Your Pantry

Even before you get started with the diet, it is important that you get the distractions out of the way. Start with your pantry.

Make sure to eliminate all the foods that don't fall within the purview of this diet. We have already seen what kinds of foods should be consumed, as part of this diet. So, start cleaning out your pantry keeping this in mind.

- Start with processed and junk foods. These are not going to do you any good! Let's get them out of the way.

- Move on to carbs next. Remember that this diet is about consuming carbs in minimal quantities. Therefore, make sure that you remove heavy carbs from the pantry. Take out the sugary foods next, for these are nothing but more carbs.

- Packaged foods should also be removed from your pantry. Many are loaded with artificial sweeteners, preservatives, and processed ingredients.

Why is this exercise important? When you remove such distracting foods from your pantry, you can worry less about deviating from your diet. ***When I meant clean your pantry, you don't have to necessarily trash it.***

If the ingredients are well within their expiration date, you can always try to give them away or donate them if they are unopened.

Go Shopping

As soon as you clear out your pantry, the next step is to restock it. Ensure that all the ingredients stocked in your pantry are Keto friendly.

To help you out here, I have put together a sample Keto shopping list, which you can use to stock your pantry. Again, this is just an illustrative list.

You can come up with your own shopping list, so long as it is designed based on the principles of this diet. Keeping only Keto friendly ingredients will definitely motivate you to stick to the diet. After all, you wouldn't want the ingredients in your pantry to rot!

Dairy

- ✓ Blue cheese
- ✓ Brie
- ✓ Butter
- ✓ Cheddar cheese
- ✓ Colby cheese
- ✓ Cottage cheese

- ✓ Cream cheese
- ✓ Crème fraiche
- ✓ Farmer's cheese
- ✓ Feta
- ✓ Greek yoghurt
- ✓ Heavy cream (40% fat)
- ✓ Homemade mayonnaise
- ✓ Mascarpone
- ✓ Mozzarella cheese
- ✓ Parmesan cheese
- ✓ Sour cream (full fat)
- ✓ Turkish yoghurt (10% fat)

Proteins and Seafood

- ✓ Bacon
- ✓ Beef roast
- ✓ Canned tuna or sardines
- ✓ Catfish
- ✓ Chicken
- ✓ Clams
- ✓ Cod
- ✓ Crabs
- ✓ Duck
- ✓ Eggs
- ✓ Goat
- ✓ Ground beef
- ✓ Ground pork
- ✓ Halibut
- ✓ Ham
- ✓ Lamb
- ✓ Mackerel
- ✓ Mussels
- ✓ Offal

- ✓ Oysters
- ✓ Pheasant
- ✓ Pork chops
- ✓ Quail
- ✓ Salmon
- ✓ Sausages
- ✓ Scallops
- ✓ Shrimp
- ✓ Snapper
- ✓ Squid
- ✓ Steak
- ✓ Tenderloin
- ✓ Trout
- ✓ Tuna
- ✓ Turkey
- ✓ Venison

Vegetables and Fruits

- ✓ Arugula
- ✓ Asparagus
- ✓ Avocados
- ✓ Bamboo shoots
- ✓ Bell peppers
- ✓ Blueberries
- ✓ Bok choy
- ✓ Broccoli
- ✓ Cabbage
- ✓ Cauliflower
- ✓ Celery
- ✓ Collard greens
- ✓ Daikon Radish
- ✓ Eggplants
- ✓ Fennel

- ✓ Green beans
- ✓ Jalapeno peppers
- ✓ Kale
- ✓ Kohlrabi
- ✓ Lemon
- ✓ Lime
- ✓ Mushrooms
- ✓ Okra
- ✓ Olives
- ✓ Onions
- ✓ Parsnip
- ✓ Peaches
- ✓ Raspberries
- ✓ Spinach
- ✓ Sprouts
- ✓ Strawberries
- ✓ Swiss chard
- ✓ Tomatoes
- ✓ Watercress
- ✓ Zucchini

Spices

- ✓ Basil
- ✓ Cayenne pepper
- ✓ Chili powder
- ✓ Cilantro
- ✓ Cinnamon
- ✓ Cumin
- ✓ Oregano
- ✓ Parsley
- ✓ Rosemary
- ✓ Thyme

Condiments, Nuts and Oils

- ✓ Almond flour
- ✓ Almonds
- ✓ Brazil nuts
- ✓ Capers
- ✓ Chia seeds meal
- ✓ Chicken stock
- ✓ Coconut oil
- ✓ Dill pickles (sugar free)
- ✓ Flaxseed meal
- ✓ Hazelnuts
- ✓ Macadamia nuts
- ✓ Mustard
- ✓ Olive oil
- ✓ Pasta sauce (with no added sugar)
- ✓ Pecans
- ✓ Pine nuts
- ✓ Pumpkin seeds
- ✓ Sesame oil (for salads)
- ✓ Sesame seeds
- ✓ Soy sauce
- ✓ Splenda
- ✓ Stevia
- ✓ Sugar free dressings
- ✓ Sunflower seeds
- ✓ Unsweetened coconut
- ✓ Vegetable oil
- ✓ Vegetable stock
- ✓ Walnuts

Baking Ingredients

✓ Plain gelatin

✓ Unsweetened cocoa powder

✓ Vanilla extract (without sugar)

✓ Whey protein powder

Beverages

✓ Black tea

✓ Broth

✓ Coffee

✓ Diet soda (try to stay away from these due to the artificial ingredients)

✓ Green tea

✓ Unsweetened almond milk

✓ Unsweetened coconut milk

✓ Water

Read the Labels Before Buying

Although I have given you a pretty exhaustive shopping list in the previous section, it is not necessary that you have such a big list with you at all times. All you need to remember, before you step out for grocery shopping, is that you should buy only those ingredients which fall under the purview of this diet. Promise yourself that you will not end up buying other grocery items which will only make you deviate from the diet.

As part of shopping, it is important that you **develop the habit of reading the labels** of the products before you add them to your cart. We always focus on the price, the quantity, the brand and other attributes like flavor, expiration date et cetera.

- One thing that most of us fail to observe is the nutrition information. We don't really pay attention to what are the nutrients present in the particular packaged product, before we add them to the cart. This is extremely crucial if you are trying to follow any diet.

- Only when you start reading nutrition information, will you be able to select only those ingredients falling under the purview of that particular diet.

If you recall, I had strictly suggested eliminating packaged and processed foods from your diet. This is because they contain a lot of added sugars and carbohydrates. Only when you start reading the labels, will you realize that the products that you have been consuming all these days are actually not good for you.

Therefore, develop the habit of reading the labels, especially the nutrition information, before you add any item to your shopping cart. This way, you can ensure that all the ingredients that you choose are within the principles of this diet.

Buy in Bulk Quantities

When you are starting a new diet, obviously there will be oppositions to change. You will be tempted to eat the things that you like, irrespective of whether they are within the purview of this diet or not.

- The initial days are extremely tricky and will have to be dealt carefully.

- If you deviate in the first week itself, the chances of you coming back to this diet are pretty slim. Even if you do come back, the resolve to stick until the end might not be there.

- Therefore, it is important that you stay focused during the first few days. Once you get past this stage, it is only going to be easier for you to follow this diet for the rest of your life.

One suggestion to help you stay on track is to buy all your grocery items in bulk quantities. There are three key benefits of buying your groceries in bulk. They are as follows:

Saves Money

When you buy your groceries in bulk, you will actually end up saving quite a bit of money. We all know that prices of large packets are always cheaper than the average sized ones. This way, as part of staying on track, you are also saving some money.

Saves Time

Typically, you would hit the grocery store at least once a week for buying your grocery items. By buying it in bulk, you are reducing the number of trips to the grocery store. We all know how going to the grocery store is such a time-consuming exercise. You can save a lot of time by reducing the number of trips to the store.

A Big Source of Motivation

When you stock your pantry with all the essential groceries in bulk quantities, the chances of you deviating from your diet are pretty slim. After all, you wouldn't want to waste so many items and deviate from the diet.

Although, you would've saved a bit of money by shopping in bulk, you would definitely not want to waste the money spent on the groceries. Every time you are hungry, you'll always be able to cook up a quick meal with the available groceries. This way, not having enough groceries is not an excuse any more for you to deviate from the diet and eat out.

Therefore, having a well-stocked pantry can be a huge motivating factor, when you are trying to follow this diet.

Stop Eating Out Before You Begin the Diet

Gone are the days when we eat out only on certain occasions. Almost, all of us end up eating out, every other day. In fact, eating home cooked meals have become such a rare thing that we don't realize what we are missing.

This habit of eating out frequently could be a major dissuading factor, when you are trying to follow any diet. This is probably because the restaurants that you go to or the fast food joints that you frequent may not always have Keto friendly ingredients or prepare their meals as per the principles of this diet.

Even though certain dishes might look Keto friendly, all the ingredients might not actually be based on the principles of this diet. In fact, if you recall, I had suggested buying sauces and flavoring agents, which don't have added sugars. There is no guarantee that these restaurants might have sourced such similar ingredients. The sauces or condiments that they use could definitely be loaded with more carbs and sugars.

Therefore, it is important that you learn to reduce the number of times you eat out, before you start this diet.

I know that it is not possible to immediately bring down the number. Take it slowly and do it gradually so that you are not starving. Ideally, you should be doing this at least a week before you start the diet. This way, you are preparing your body to certain dietary changes.

Previously, if you were eating out 10 times a week, try bringing it down to six. As and when you go through the diet, you can bring the instances down to an even smaller number. By doing this, you are also preparing your mind for following this diet. You will be less tempted to go out and eat, when you are following the diet, if you started implementing this.

Irrespective of you following any diet, this conscious decision of bringing down the number of times that you eat outside is always going to benefit you in the long run.

- One important reason why most of us face obesity and other lifestyle related disorders is because of the drastic increase in the number of meals that we consume outside our home every day.

- Just as in the case of shopping, not all of us actually pay attention to the ingredients being used in those dishes.

There are new studies emerging every other day, which keep reiterating the harmful nature of added preservatives and artificial flavoring agents. Therefore, make sure that you implement this habit, irrespective of whether you are following any diet or not.

Keep a Tab on the Protein Content

It's extremely important that you remember that **this is not a high-protein diet**. This is a high-fat diet and you are required to consume only just enough protein. Keep this in mind when you are buying your groceries or eating out or preparing your meals. Make sure that the protein content in your meals is not too high.

If it is indeed high, you will end up not losing any weight. **When you consume too much protein, your body automatically starts secreting insulin.** The rate at which your body burns the fat deposited is also affected and you would actually require a lot of time to lose weight.

When you are following a diet and when you can't see any immediate results, you will definitely be discouraged to stick to it or follow it again. Therefore, it is crucial that you don't include protein in your meals in high quantities.

Consume Root Vegetables in Minimal Quantities

While there is not much restriction on the consumption of vegetables and fruit, you really need to keep an eye on the intake of root vegetables. This is because root vegetables are loaded with sugar and carbohydrates.

- Since the intent of this diet is to consume carbohydrates in minimum quantities, you should keep an eye out for these vegetables. Although, I have included them in the grocery list, make sure that you buy them only in small quantities.

- Another thing about root vegetables is that most of them contain starch, which is just more carbohydrates. Therefore, be mindful about the inclusion of root vegetables, as part of your diet.

Formulate Your Own Support Group

As I have mentioned already, the initial days of the diet are extremely tricky. You would be tempted to deviate at the first chance you get. If you are sure that you don't have a strong resolve, there is nothing wrong in asking for the support of others to help you through this journey.

It is important that you come up with your own support group of friends and family, before you even begin this diet. The reason why I am insisting on coming up with your support group is because it has several benefits.

Some of the key benefits of having your own support group are as follows:

No More Peer Pressure

The reason why most people deviate from their diet plans is because of peer pressure. I understand that it can be extremely difficult to turn down the invitation of a friend to go out for dinner, especially if that friend is really persuasive. It is again not possible to bail out of most outings, under the pretext of following a diet.

Therefore, it is important that you keep your family and friends in the loop about your dieting goals. Take the time and explain to them why this diet is important to you. Explain the objective behind following the diet.

For example, if the intention behind following this diet is to lose weight and minimize your risk factors for several lifestyle related disorders, explain it in greater detail to them. Once you have their support, the chances of them asking you to deviate from your diet and come out with them for dinners or outings would be minimal.

Therefore, with peer pressure out of the way, the number of times you would actually deviate from the diet will be very minimal.

Constant Motivation

When you lack the motivation to stick to the diet, you can always take the help of family or friends to follow through. Once you have decided on your meal plan, make sure that you share it with your friends or family members. This way, they can follow up, as and when necessary, and make sure that you stick to the plan.

Of course, you can take the help of reminders. But, a snooze button is all you need to push a reminder out of the way. The same cannot be said for a human reminder. You will not be able to avoid their reminders for too long.

If you are able to successfully implement the meal plan in the first few days, thanks to the support, then you would be able to take it forward from there, on your own. Therefore, the higher number of people you have on board, the greater the motivation will be!

When you have the support of your family and friends, following this diet will not seem like a daunting task after all. In fact, you could also encourage them to follow this diet along with you. This way, you will have somebody else sharing this journey with you and you will think twice before you deviate.

Incorporating Changes

If you're going to be incorporating changes to your dietary habits and if it is going to impact the other members in your family, it is important that they are kept in the loop about it.

- For example, if your mom has to take extra precautions while preparing meals at home, you will need to tell her the exact specifications of the diet. Otherwise, she might end up missing the principles of the diet.

- Another thing about implementing a diet is that it is extra work. Now, if your mom has to prepare an extra set of meals, just for you, it is important that you let her know the reason behind this diet and get her support. If you have her buy-in, following the diet is not going to be a daunting task at all.

This is why it is important that you come up with your own support system. Every time you try to deviate from the plan, there will always be somebody trying to back you up and push you in the right direction. Staying on track is important if you want to enjoy the benefits of any diet plan. It is not wise that you start off with a diet and then just stop it midway. Only if you follow it consistently, will you be able to enjoy the long-term benefits of the diet.

Join Social Groups

I have already stressed on the importance of having your own support system, before you start any diet. It is important that you get the support of your family and friends. It is equally important that you connect with other people following the same diet. This is because, when you start a diet, your body will obviously oppose it. You might have some reactions to a certain diet or you might have tons of questions about implementing a certain diet.

Of course, you can always look it up online. But, it is not the same as getting the input from another person, who has successfully implemented this diet. While you can always take the help of a professional dietician, before you implement the diet, it is going to benefit you in more than one way, if you join social groups formed for people following this diet. Let's look at some of the key benefits of joining these forums.

- You will get an opportunity to interact with people from all walks of life, who are implementing this diet. You will be able to get specific feedback and input from them, with respect to following the diets. These insights will help you design your meal plan in such a way that you are addressing all your allergies and your preferences in the best manner possible.

- These social forums also contain suggestions for implementing this diet effectively. Each person would have shared his own success story, which could be useful, when you are trying to implement this diet. There could be specific tips, which will help you get started and follow this diet properly.
- The beauty about these social forums is that people get to share the success stories. When they receive recognition from the rest of the members, they feel motivated to keep going. As a beginner, you need every bit of motivation to hold onto this diet. When you share your success story, you will really feel good about yourself and the progress that you have made. The recognition that you get by doing so, will help you stay motivated enough to follow this diet.
- If you want to stay updated about the key findings pertaining to this diet, the best way to do so is to be part of these forums. People tend to share the latest research studies surrounding this diet and also the results of such studies. You will be able to be abreast of all the latest studies regarding this diet and this will also reassure you that you are doing the right thing by following this diet.
- The social groups are not just for posting the good things. People often share the stories of how they deviated from the diet and what it looked like for them to get back on track. These forums can provide you the opportunity of learning from others' mistakes. Therefore, when you are trying to implement this diet, you can plan your schedule and meal plan in such a way that you avoid common pitfalls.
- More than your family member or friend trying to motivate you, you would feel more motivated if a person in the social group pushed you to follow this

diet. This is because the person advising you is going through the same journey as you and would be able to relate to you better than your family or friends, who are not following this diet.

- We tend to take the counsel of people, who have already walked the path, seriously. Therefore, if you are thinking about deviating from this diet, these social forums can be a source of support to you.

Maintain a Food Journal

Getting into the habit of maintaining a food journal will actually help you in implementing any diet in an effective manner. As I said before, we don't really pay attention to what we eat, let alone worry about the harmful nature of the ingredients we are consuming. Even before you implement this diet, it is important that you learn to maintain a food journal. When you start doing this, you will be more aware about your dietary habits.

- Record every meal that you consume, along with nutrition information. Now, it might not be possible to predict the nutrition value of all meals accurately, especially if you are eating them outside.

- As long as you put in an estimated figure, you are good to go. After recording all entries for a week, take a look at the journal. You will be able to assess in what quantities you have been consuming of various nutrients.

- For instance, you will be able to assess if you have been following a high carb diet, based on these entries. This information will give you an insight on what is required to implement the keto diet effectively.

- For example, if you are already following a high-fat and high-carb diet, you need to focus only on the reduction of the carbs intake.

- Maintaining a food journal will help you gain specific insights into your dietary habits and come up with a proper plan for implementing the Keto diet.

The practice of maintaining a journal will also help you in sticking to the diet. For instance, if you have to record every entry in your journal, you would think twice before you deviate from the diet. When you record all your meals in a diligent manner, you will also be able to quickly catch any deviation and make sure that you compensate for it in the upcoming meals.

- For example, if you realize that you have consumed more carbs in your breakfast, you can skip carbs for the rest of the meals and focus only on fat and protein. This way, you are still sticking to the principles of your diet, although you should try to maintain as much consistency as possible.

Having a journal will also help you keep track of your progress. Keeping track of your progress is essential to tweak your diet plan accordingly.

- For instance, if you realize that you are struggling to stick to the diet, you can identify the distracting factors and come up with ways to deal with them. On the other hand, if you realize that you are making good progress, you will actually feel motivated to continue following this diet.

Managing Social Outings

I know that it is not possible to always stay indoors and just eat home cooked meals. At some point in time, you will have to accept invitations to social outings. However, it is important that you stick to your diet, no matter what. While this can be tricky, it is not impossible. A couple of tips to help you come out of these social meetings, without deviating from your diet plan, are as follows:

Eat Before You Go Out

If you were not sure about the menu at the meeting, it would do you good if you didn't eat out much. It is not possible for you to find only keto friendly items at the dinner. Therefore, the best way to eat less out is by actually eating at home before you venture out. I know this might sound crazy, but trust me you will feel good about not deviating from your diet!

Refuse the Menu Card

If you know which restaurant you are going to, you can actually look up the menu online before you go out. Try to identify those items which are based on the principles of this diet. Choose the dish that you want to eat. When you reach the restaurant, decline the menu card and order the dish that you have chosen. This way, the odds of you getting tempted by other items on the menu and ordering something, which is not permissible under your diet, are very low.

Let Your Host Know Your Preference

If you are being invited to a friend or colleague's house for dinner, do let them know that you are dieting and you would like to eat light. By informing them upfront, you are giving them an opportunity to have a Keto-friendly dish on the menu. If that were not possible, at least you won't come across as a rude person, who keeps turning down every dish at the table.

This way, you will not feel pressured to eat any dish, which is not keto friendly.

Keep Your Body Hydrated

When you are introducing changes to your dietary habits, it is important that you take necessary precautions. One such precaution is to keep your body hydrated at all times. Consuming enough fluids throughout the day will actually help in sustaining your energy levels as well.

It will also aid in the digestion process. Another advantage of drinking lots of water is that it helps in fat metabolism. Thus, you are accelerating the weight loss by keeping your body sufficiently hydrated. Make sure to drink at least 6 to 8 glasses of water every day. You can also opt for other juices, so long as they are not loaded with sugar.

Consume Chicken Broth

As we have already seen in the previous chapter, the sodium and potassium content present in your kidneys get flushed out of the body, when you are following this diet. This could result in possible electrolyte imbalances. These imbalances could affect your blood pressure levels as well.

Therefore, it is important that you maintain a balance, when it comes to the electrolyte levels in your body. Instead of adding more salt to your food, you can opt to include chicken broth as part of your meals. Chicken broth is capable of improving your electrolyte levels in a jiffy. If you don't have the time to incorporate it as part of a recipe, you could just heat it and drink it out of a cup!

Come Up with a Suitable Reward System

To keep you motivated to stay on track, you need to come up with your own reward system. Some of the key benefits of having a reward system in place are as follows:

- You don't have to rely on others to motivate you to stay on track. You will be motivated automatically by your own reward system and that is enough to help you stay on track.
- When you realize that there is a reward for staying on track the entire week, you will think twice before deviating from your diet. The initial few days of dieting could be quite challenging and you could always use some extra motivation. Having a reward system will help you with that!

However, there are certain ground rules that you need to put in place, before you design your reward system. Let's look at some of those rules. Again, these are pretty illustrative in nature. You can tweak them as you please.

Set Tangible Goals First

Even before you come up with a reward, you need to be clear about your goals. Take some time in setting your dieting goals. Don't go overboard and come up with unrealistic goals. The goals that you set should be measurable, practical and achievable.

- For example, you can come up with a goal of cooking all your meals for one week. Try to go for short-term goals, as they can provide you a specific sense of direction. Trust me when I say that this sense of direction will help you in implementing your diet in an effective manner.

Come Up with Appropriate Rewards

Rewards can be quite tricky and you need to design your reward system with care. You will have to choose the quantum of the reward, based on the amount of effort involved.

- For example, if you are someone who lives on junk foods, it might be difficult for you to give it up altogether from tomorrow. Therefore, a realistic goal would be to bring down the number of days you eat junk foods from 7 to 4. You need to choose a suitable reward for the effort involved in actually cutting down the intake of junk foods by half.

- If your reward is too lavish, you will be too occupied with it and lose track of the diet. On the other hand, if your reward is not sufficient, you will not be motivated to stick to the diet. Therefore, choosing the right reward is absolutely crucial, if you want to stay motivated. Don't be in a hurry. Take some time and also the help of another individual to come up with an unbiased reward system.

Time Your Rewards Properly

If you want to derive motivation from having a reward system, it is imperative that you decide on the timing of the rewards as well. If you are trying to start this diet for the first time, you have to make sure that your rewards are timely so that you don't deviate from the diet at the first opportunity that presents itself.

If your reward is not immediate, you will not bother sticking to the principles of this diet. Therefore, try to reward yourself as soon as practically possible. At the same time, don't reward yourself in anticipation of meeting your goals. That will never do you any good.

Rewards Should be in Line with the Diet

The whole point of having a reward system in the first place is to ensure that you follow the diet. Therefore, you should choose your rewards in such a way that it does not contradict your dieting efforts. For instance, you can't choose a heavy carb meal as a reward for following the diet successfully for a week. Therefore, come up with healthy rewards.

These are just illustrative ground rules for your reward system. As I mentioned before, it is important that you spend some time in carefully designing your reward system, for it will help you implement the diet in an effective manner.

In fact, the time that you spend upfront in designing your reward system will actually save you the time that you would end up using looking for some kind of motivation to stick to the diet. If you deviate, it's going to take even more time to get back on track.

Be Consistent

When it comes to any diet, consistency is extremely crucial. While this is a high fat, low-carb diet, it doesn't mean that you can eat fatty foods for two meals of the day and carb-rich foods for the third meal. You will have to ensure that each meal you consume is as balanced as possible. Try to achieve the desired ratio of these nutrients in every meal.

Of course, there might be negligible deviations, here and there. But that is fine. What's important is that you strive to achieve consistency with all your meals. The more consistent you are, the sooner you will be able to reap the benefits of this diet. Your body will take less time to adjust to this diet, if you are consistent in your efforts.

Therefore, have a clear understanding of the diet before you even get started and ensure consistency as you go along.

Track Your Progress

There is no point in coming up with a meal plan or dieting goals, if you are not planning to track your progress. Only when you actually track your progress, will you be able to see how effectively you are able to implement the diet and tackle any deviations in an appropriate manner. Here's why tracking your progress is crucial:

- You will be able to identify when you are deviating. This awareness can help you avoid such pitfalls in the future. You can look up similar stories in social forums and see how those individuals had overcome their challenges.
- You will be able to identify those tips/practices, which are working for you. You can continue implementing them to stick to your diet and also share your story for the others to learn from your best practice.
- You will be able to assess what is needed to achieve your dieting goal, in the light of changing circumstances. For example, your goal is to lose 4 pounds at least this month. When you review your progress, you realize that you are nowhere near to achieving this mark. You can reevaluate your diet plan to see any slippages. You can also consider increasing your exercise time, for ensuring that you achieve this dieting goal.
- When you realize that you are on track, it could be a huge motivating factor for you to stick to the diet.

As I said, unless you know your progress, you will not be able to figure out if you are effectively implementing your diet or not. Here are some tips for helping you track your progress:

- Make use of your food journal. This can actually help you get a thorough understanding of your dietary habits and help you track if you are sticking to the diet or not.
- If you are not sure about your abilities to gauge your progress, you can take the help of a friend or family member. You can ask them to review your food journal and see how well you have fared.
- Take the help of reminders. This way, you will not miss your periodical reviews. Take some time in deciding the frequency of these reviews. For instance, if you are someone with a strong resolve, you don't have to set up too frequent reviews. This is because you are generally confident of sticking to the diet.
- On the other hand, if you are sure that you are prone to distractions and you would easily deviate from the diet plan, make sure that your reviews are frequent. This way, you can immediately catch any deviation and take corrective action.

Don't Exercise During the First Two Weeks

As I already mentioned, there will be certain oppositions from your body, when you are trying to implement any changes to your dietary habits. Further, when your body is trying to derive energy from burning the fats, it will be at its tired state. The least you can do is to not exert yourself more, until your body gets accustomed to the low carb intake.

By reducing the carbs intake, you are actually cutting down the energy source of your body. Therefore, it is important that you learn to conserve your energy as much as possible. Unless you are an athlete, you should abstain from any form of exercising for at least two weeks. If you follow this diet, without any deviations, these two weeks should be sufficient time for your body to start relying on the fat content in different parts of your body for energy.

Take it easy and don't be in a hurry to try out everything to lose weight quickly. You will only end up burning yourself out!

Cook Your Own Meals

I know that cooking can be quite a daunting task, if you don't really have an idea what you are cooking. But, when you cook your own meals, you can be sure that you are including keto friendly ingredients, as part of your cooking. You can also ensure that you are being consistent in your efforts to implement this diet. Some tips to help you take up cooking are as follows:

- Plan your meals in advance. This way, you can ensure that you have all the grocery items required for your meals. When you plan your meals in advance, you will end up visualizing them. This will also motivate you to cook them!
- Do all the prep work overnight. Preparing the ingredients tends to take more time than the cooking itself. Therefore, before you hit the bed, prepare the ingredients for the next day's meals. This way, you will only have to spend few minutes in the kitchen to quickly whip up a meal.
- Cook smartly. Make use of appliances like slow cooker or a pressure cooker, which will require minimal supervision. All you need to do is throw in the ingredients and go about your daily routine. The food will get cooked in its own time and you don't have to stand next to the counter at all times.
- To begin with, try cooking at least one meal per day. Commit to trying out at least one new recipe a day.

This will keep you motivated over the long run, at least until you pick up the interest to cook.

To help you get started, I have also provided several exciting recipes in the upcoming chapters. You can try out these recipes, to begin with, until you get a grasp over cooking!

Be Patient and Learn to Move On

When you are implementing this diet, take only one step at a time. This is true for implementing any diet plan for that matter. If you really want to stay motivated to follow the diet, you will have to introduce only incremental changes, to begin with. Don't be in a hurry to implement this diet. When you hurry, it might appear that you have actually implemented your diet properly. However, it will backfire on you and you will deviate from the diet. Therefore, make one change at a time to the way you eat.

There will obviously some deviations, during the initial few weeks of starting the diet. Don't hold on to these mistakes for too long. Don't be hard on yourself either. When you realize that you have deviated from the diet, identify the root cause and come up with a way to overcome it, instead of sulking about deviating. I

t's never too late to get back on track. So, don't let your mistakes/deviations stop you from following this diet. Try implementing this diet from tomorrow, with renewed energy. Don't think that your deviations occur because your diet is too strict. As I said before, this diet is one of the least restrictive ones, where you still get to hold on to your favorite fatty foods. Therefore, it is only a matter of your mindset before you can get your act straight and resume the diet.

I am sure that you found these tips useful. Be patient and remember to be consistent with your efforts. You should be able to successfully implement and stick to this diet, in due course.

Chapter Four: Ketogenic Condiment Recipes

Zero Carb Mayonnaise

Serves: 32 servings of 1 tablespoon each

Nutritional values per serving: 1 tablespoon

Calories – 95, Fat – 11 g, Carbohydrates – 0 g, Protein – 0 g

Ingredients:

- 2 egg yolks, at room temperature
- 2 tablespoons lemon juice
- 6 tablespoons apple cider vinegar
- ½ teaspoon salt or to taste
- ½ teaspoon garlic powder
- 1 ½ cups avocado oil
- ½ teaspoon paprika

Method:

1. Add all the ingredients into a blender and blend until creamy and smooth.
2. Pour into a glass jar. Fasten the lid and refrigerate until use.

5 Minute Keto Pesto

Serves: 12 servings of 1 tablespoon each

Nutritional values per serving: 1 tablespoon

Calories – 79, Fat – 8.09 g, Carbohydrates – 0.84 g, Protein – 1.22 g

Ingredients:

- ¾ cup fresh basil
- 6 tablespoons Parmesan cheese, grated
- ½ teaspoon garlic, minced
- 1 teaspoon tomato paste
- 3 tablespoons pine nuts, toasted
- 1/3 cup olive oil
- Salt to taste
- Pepper to taste

Method:

1. Add all the ingredients except oil into a blender and blend until smooth.
2. With the motor running, pour the oil in a thin stream through the feeder tube of the blender jar.
3. Transfer into a glass jar. Fasten the lid. Refrigerate until use.

Caesar Dressing

Serves: 16 servings of 1 tablespoon each

Nutritional values per serving:

Calories – 100.39, Fat – 10.74 g, Carbohydrates – 0.56 g, Protein – 0.54 g

Ingredients:

- 6 cloves garlic, finely minced
- 2 teaspoons Worcestershire sauce
- 3 teaspoons Dijon mustard
- Salt to taste
- Pepper to taste
- 3 teaspoons anchovy paste
- 4 tablespoons fresh lemon juice
- 1 ½ cups mayonnaise

Method:

1. Add all the ingredients into a bowl and whisk until well combined.
2. Transfer into a glass jar. Fasten the lid. Refrigerate until use.

Chia Seed and Strawberry Jam

Serves: 10 servings of 1 tablespoon each

Nutritional values per serving: 1 tablespoon

Calories – 9.65, Fat – 0.58 g, Carbohydrates – 1.42 g, Protein – 0.35 g

Ingredients:

- 4 ounces fresh strawberries, chopped
- 1 tablespoon chia seeds
- 2 tablespoons stevia, powdered
- 2 tablespoons water

Method:

1. Add strawberries into a small pan. Place the pan over medium heat.
2. Add stevia and stir. In a while the strawberries will begin to release its juices. Mash the strawberries with a potato masher.
3. Simmer until slightly thick. Add chia seeds and cook for a couple of minutes.
4. Turn off the heat. Let it cool for a while.
5. Transfer into a glass jar. Fasten the lid. Refrigerate until use.

Guacamole

Serves: 16 servings of 1 tablespoon each

Nutritional values per serving: 1 tablespoon

Calories – 16.56, Fat – 1.41 g, Carbohydrates – 1.11g, Protein – 0.23 g

Ingredients:

- 1 whole Hass avocados, peeled, seeded, mashed with a fork
- 2 tablespoons lime juice
- 1 tablespoon pre-made salsa
- 1 small red onion, finely chopped
- ½ teaspoon sea salt
- ½ cup fresh cilantro, finely chopped
- 1 jalapeno pepper, finely sliced
- Black pepper powder to taste

Method:

1. Mix together all the ingredients in a bowl.
2. Cover and chill until use.

Chive Egg Dip

Serves: 24 servings of 2 tablespoons each

Nutritional values per serving: 2 tablespoons

Calories – 58, Fat – 5 g, Carbohydrates – 1 g, Protein – 2 g

Ingredients:

- 4 eggs, hard boiled, coarsely chopped
- 2 teaspoons Dijon mustard or prepared mustard
- ¼ cup mayonnaise
- ½ teaspoon garlic powder (optional)
- 4 packages (3 ounces each) cream cheese, softened
- ½ cup fresh chives, minced
- 2 teaspoons Worcestershire sauce
- Sea salt to taste
- Pepper powder to taste
- ½ cup milk

Method:

1. Add all the ingredients except chives to a blender and blend until smooth.
2. Transfer into a bowl. Add chives and stir.
3. Cover and chill until use.

Egg Fast Alfredo Sauce

Serves: 10 servings of 1 tablespoon each

Nutritional values per serving: 1 tablespoon

Calories – 48, Fat – 5 g, Carbohydrates – 0.4 g, Protein – 1 g

Ingredients:

- 2 ounces cream cheese, softened
- ½ teaspoon granulated garlic
- 2 tablespoons unsalted butter
- A large pinch ground nutmeg
- 4 tablespoons water
- Freshly ground pepper to taste
- Salt to taste
- 3 tablespoons Parmesan cheese, grated
- A handful fresh basil or Italian parsley, chopped (optional)

Method:

1. Add cream cheese, pepper, water and garlic into a microwave safe bowl.
2. Microwave on High for 12-15 seconds.
3. Remove the bowl from the microwave. Add butter and stir until butter melts.
4. Add rest of the ingredients and stir.
5. Serve.

Chapter Five: Ketogenic Breakfast Recipes

Cheese and Ham Waffles

Serves: 2

Nutritional values per serving:

Calories – 626, Fat – 48 g, Carbohydrates – 1 g, Protein – 45 g

Ingredients:

- 2 scoops unflavored whey protein powder
- 4 large eggs
- 6 tablespoons melted butter
- 1 tablespoon baking powder
- ½ teaspoon sea salt
- 1 ounce cheddar cheese, finely grated
- Paprika
- 1 ounce ham steak (try to buy ham without nitrates), chopped finely
- Fresh basil, finely chopped

Method:

1. Separate 2 eggs into yolks and whites into 2 mixing bowls.
2. Add the baking powder, sea salt, protein powder and melted butter to the bowl containing the egg yolks. Whisk well until well combined.
3. Add grated cheese and chopped ham to the egg yolk mixture. Fold gently.

4. Add a pinch of salt to the bowl containing the egg whites and whisk with the help of an electric hand mixer until stiff peaks form.

5. Mix half the whites mixture with the egg yolk mixture and fold well. Be extremely gentle when you are folding in the egg whites, to make sure that the yolks don't deflate.

6. Once the egg yolks have aerated enough, add rest of the whites and fold gently. Your batter is now ready.

7. Grease the waffle maker and let it preheat. Take about ¼ cup of the batter and add it to the waffle maker. Cook the waffles, as per the instructions of the manufacturer. The waffles need around 3 to 4 minutes to turn golden, over a medium heat.

8. Repeat the above step with rest of the batter to make more waffles.

9. As the waffles are cooking, cook 2 of the eggs, two sunny sides up.

10. Divide the cooked waffles between two serving plate.

11. Arrange an egg on top of each waffle stack. Sprinkle some paprika and chopped basil over the egg.

12. Serve warm.

Bacon, Cheese and Egg Cups

Serves: 12

Nutritional values per serving:

Calories – 101, Fat – 7 g, Carbohydrates – 1 g, Protein – 8 g

Ingredients:

- 1/3 cup cheddar cheese, finely shredded
- Salt to taste
- Pepper to taste
- 12 strips bacon (try to buy bacon naturally preserved and cured without nitrates)
- 12 large eggs
- ½ cup of frozen spinach, thawed and drained well
- Olive oil to grease

Method:

1. Preheat the oven to 400° F.
2. Place a pan over medium heat. Add the bacon strips and fry it for few minutes. Place the strips on a plate that is lined with paper towels.
3. Grease a 12-cup muffin pan with olive oil.
4. Add one bacon slice to each cup and press them down in such a way that they stick up on either side of the cups.
5. Add the eggs into a large bowl and beat them gently.
6. Before adding the spinach to the eggs, make sure that the leaves are not wet. Make use of a paper towel to drain off any water. Add the spinach leaves to the eggs and stir well.

7. Divide the mixture equally among the muffin cups. The mixture should fill up only about ¾th of the cup.
8. Divide the shredded cheese among the muffin cups. Season each cup with salt and pepper.
9. Place the muffin cups in the oven and bake for around 15 minutes.
10. When done, cool slightly. Run a knife around the edges cup and invert on to a plate.
11. Transfer into an airtight container and refrigerate until use. Heat before serving.

Apple and Brie Crepes

Serves: 4

Nutritional values per serving:

Calories – 411, Fat – 37 g, Carbohydrates – 6 g, Protein – 14 g

Ingredients:

For the batter:

- 4 large eggs
- ¼ teaspoon of sea salt
- 4 ounces of cream cheese
- ½ teaspoon of baking soda

For the topping:

- ¼ teaspoon of cinnamon
- 2 ounces of chopped pecans
- 4 ounces of brie cheese, thinly sliced
- 1 tablespoon of unsalted butter
- Fresh mint leaves, for garnish
- 1 small apple, cut into slices

Method:

1. To make crème batter: Add the eggs, cream cheese, sea salt and baking soda into a blender and blend until smooth.
2. Place a nonstick pan over medium heat and add a little of the unsalted butter to it. Let the butter melt.
3. Take some of the batter and spread it on the pan. Cook the batter for around 2 to 3 minutes, until the top becomes dry and the bottom is golden brown. Flip and cook the other side for few more seconds.

4. Repeat with the remaining batter to make 11 more crepes.
5. Add the rest of the butter to a small pan and add the chopped pecans to it. Toast the pecans, until they turn fragrant.
6. Sprinkle the cinnamon on top of the pecans and mix well. Remove it from the heat and keep it aside.
7. Divide the apple slices and cheese slices among the 12 crepes.
8. Add the toasted pecan mix to each crepe. Garnish with mint leaves and serve warm.

Zucchini and Chicken Quiche

Serves: 10

Nutritional values per serving:

Calories – 311, Fat – 25 g, Carbohydrates – 4 g, Protein – 18 g

Ingredients:

For the crust:

- 2 tablespoons of coconut oil
- 1 large egg
- 2 cups almond flour
- 1 pinch of sea salt

For the filling:

- 1 to 2 medium zucchinis, finely grated
- 6 large eggs
- 1 teaspoon fennel seed
- ½ cup heavy cream
- 1 teaspoon dried oregano
- 1 teaspoon salt
- 1 pound ground chicken
- ½ teaspoon black pepper

Method:

1. Preheat the oven to 350° F.
2. To make crust: Add the sea salt and almond flour into the food processor bowl and pulse well.
3. Add the egg and coconut oil to the processor next and pulse. Keep pulsing until you get dough in the shape of a ball. Remove from the processor and keep it aside.
4. Take a 9-inch pie dish and grease it well. Spread the crust dough evenly inside the pie dish.

5. Place a large skillet over medium heat. Add the ground chicken and cook until brown. Remove from the heat and keep it aside.
6. Add eggs into a large bowl and whisk until smooth.
7. Add the spices and cream to the bowl and mix well.
8. Add the cooked chicken and grated zucchini and mix well.
9. Add the filling to the crust in the pie dish. Spread it evenly.
10. Bake for 30 to 40 minutes or until done.
11. Slice into thin wedges and serve warm!

Blueberry Coconut Porridge

Serves: 2

Nutritional values per serving:

Calories – 405, Fat – 34 g, Carbohydrates – 8 g, Protein – 10 g

Ingredients:

For the porridge:

- ¼ cup ground flaxseed
- 1 cup almond milk
- 1 pinch salt
- ¼ cup coconut flour
- 1 teaspoon vanilla extract
- 1 teaspoon cinnamon
- 10 drops liquid stevia

For the toppings:

- 2 ounces blueberries
- 2 tablespoons butter
- 1 ounces shaved coconut
- 2 tablespoons pumpkin seeds

Method:

1. Add the almond milk to a pan and heat it over a low heat.
2. Add the coconut flour, salt, flaxseed and cinnamon to the pan and whisk well. Make sure that there are no lumps in the mixture.
3. In a while it will start bubbling. Add in the vanilla extract and liquid stevia. Mix well. Stir constantly.

4. Once the mixture has reached the desired consistency, remove it from the heat.
5. Stir in the blueberries, pumpkin seeds, butter and shaved coconut.
6. Serve.

Lemon Poppy Seed Pancakes

Serves: 4

Nutritional values per serving:

Calories – 355, Fat – 26 g, Carbohydrates – 6.5 g, Protein – 23 g

Ingredients:

For the pancakes:

- 6 large eggs
- 13 ounces whole milk ricotta cheese
- Juice from 2 large lemons
- ¼ teaspoon sea salt
- 1 ½ teaspoons baking powder
- 1 ½ teaspoons vanilla extract
- Zest from 2 large lemons
- ½ cup almond flour
- 25 drops liquid stevia
- 1 ½ tablespoons poppy seeds

For the lemon glaze:

- Juice from ½ a lemon
- ½ cup powdered stevia
- 1 splash almond milk

Method:

1. Add the lemon juice, zest, vanilla extract, liquid stevia and eggs into food processor bowl and blend well.
2. Add the sea salt, baking powder, almond flour, and ricotta cheese and poppy seeds to the food processor and pulse until well combined.

3. Place a large griddle over a medium heat and heat it. Ladle some of the batter and spread it over the griddle. Allow the pancake to cook until the underside is golden brown and dry on the top.
4. Flip the pancake and allow the other side to cook for another 2 minutes.
5. Repeat the above 2 steps with rest of the batter to make more pancakes.
6. Transfer the cooked pancakes onto serving plates.
7. Add the powdered stevia, almond milk and lemon juice to a small bowl. Stir well to achieve a glaze like consistency.
8. Pour the glaze over the pancakes and serve immediately.

Feta & Pesto Omelet

Serves: 2

Nutritional values per serving: Without serving option

Calories – 570, Fat – 46 g, Carbohydrates – 2.5 g, Protein – 30 g

Ingredients:

- 2 tablespoons butter
- 2 tablespoons heavy cream
- 2 tablespoons pesto
- Pepper to taste
- Salt to taste
- 6 eggs
- 2 ounces feta cheese
- Chopped basil to garnish

Method:

1. Add eggs and cream into a bowl. Whisk well.

2. Place a skillet over medium heat. Add 1-tablespoon butter. When butter melts, pour half the egg mixture into it.
3. When the omelet is nearly done, spread 1-tablespoon pesto on one half of the omelet. Sprinkle half the feta cheese over the pesto. Fold the other half of the omelet over it.
4. Cook until cheese melts and the omelet is cooked well.
5. Sprinkle some more feta on top if desired. Garnish with basil and serve with fresh, chopped tomatoes.
6. Repeat steps 2-5 to make the second omelet.

Scramble

Nutritional values per serving:

Calories – 444, Fat – 35 g, Carbohydrates – 2 g, Protein – 25 g

Ingredients:

- 12 eggs
- 4 tablespoons sour cream
- 8 strips bacon
- 1 teaspoon garlic powder
- ½ teaspoon pepper or to taste
- 1 teaspoon onion powder
- ½ teaspoon paprika
- 4 tablespoons butter
- 4 green onions, thinly sliced
- 1 teaspoon salt or to taste

Method:

1. Place a skillet over medium heat. Add bacon and cook until crisp. Remove with a slotted spoon and place on a plate that is lined with paper towels. Set aside.
2. Take a nonstick skillet and break the eggs into it. Add butter and do not whisk the eggs.
3. Place the skillet over medium high heat. Start stirring with a spatula.
4. Stir constantly. Keep taking the skillet off heat every few minutes and continue stirring.
5. When the eggs are cooked as per your desire, turn off the heat.
6. Add rest of the ingredients except bacon and mix well.
7. Sprinkle bacon on top and serve.

Blackberry Egg Bake

Serves: 10

Nutritional values per serving:

Calories – 144, Fat – 10 g, Net Carbohydrates – 2 g, Protein – 8.5 g

Ingredients:

- 10 large eggs
- 6 tablespoons coconut flour
- ½ teaspoon vanilla extract
- Zest of an orange, grated
- 1 cup fresh blackberries
- 2 tablespoons butter, melted
- 2 teaspoons fresh ginger, grated
- 2/3 teaspoon fine sea salt
- 2 teaspoons fresh rosemary

Method:

1. Add eggs, coconut flour, vanilla, orange zest, butter, ginger and salt into a blender and blend until smooth.
2. Add rosemary and pulse until well mixed.
3. Take 8 ramekins and pour the batter equally into the ramekins. Place the ramekins on a baking sheet.
4. Bake in a preheated oven 350° F for 15-20 minutes. Mixture may puff up while baking which is perfectly normal.
5. Remove from the oven and cool for a while.
6. Serve warm.

Creamy Cauliflower and Ground Beef Skillet

Serves: 2

Nutritional values per serving:

Calories – 688, Fat – 52.2 g, Carbohydrates – 16.1 g, Protein – 38 g

Ingredients:

- 1 tablespoon ghee
- 1 clove garlic, chopped
- ½ pound lean ground beef
- Freshly cracked pepper to taste
- ¼ cup mayonnaise + 2 tablespoons to drizzle
- 2 tablespoons toasted sunflower seed butter
- ½ teaspoon fish sauce
- 2 large eggs
- ¼ ripe avocado, peeled, diced
- ½ tablespoon apple cider vinegar
- 2 tablespoons chopped onions
- 2 jalapeños peppers, sliced, divided
- ½ teaspoon Himalayan salt
- ½ pound grated cauliflower
- ¼ cup water
- ½ tablespoon coconut aminos
- ½ teaspoon ground cumin
- A handful fresh parsley, chopped

Method:

1. Place a cast iron skillet or any other heavy bottomed skillet over medium high heat.
2. Add ghee. When it melts, add onion, garlic and half the jalapeño pepper slices and sauté for a few minutes until onions are translucent.

3. Stir in beef, pepper and salt and sauté until beef is not pink any more.
4. Reduce heat to medium low and add cauliflower and sauté for a couple of minutes.
5. Add ¼ cup mayonnaise, sun butter, water, coconut aminos, cumin and fish sauce into a small bowl and mix well. Pour into the skillet and mix well. Sauté for a few minutes until the mixture is slightly dry.
6. Turn off the heat. Make 2 cavities in the mixture. Crack an egg into each of the cavity. Season with salt and pepper. Sprinkle the remaining jalapeños pepper slices over it.
7. Transfer the skillet into a preheated oven. Broil for 8-10 minutes until the eggs are cooked as per your liking.
8. Meanwhile, make the sauce as follows: Mix together in a bowl, 2 tablespoons mayonnaise and apple cider vinegar. Drizzle over the skillet.
9. Top with avocado and parsley and serve.

...ing Meatloaf

Serves: 8

Nutritional values per serving:

Calories –682, Fat –56 g, Carbohydrates –5 g, Protein –38 g

Ingredients:

- 12 large eggs
- ½ yellow onion, chopped
- 2 cups cheddar cheese, shredded
- 2 pounds bulk sweet Italian sausage or breakfast sausage
- 8 ounces cream cheese, at room temperature, divided
- 4 tablespoons scallions
- Melted ghee to grease

Method:

1. Grease a loaf pan with ghee and set aside.
2. Add eggs into a bowl and beat it lightly. Add onion, sausage and half the cream cheese into it and mix until well combined.
3. Transfer the mixture into the prepared loaf pan.
4. Bake in a preheated oven at 375° F for about 25-30 minutes or until firm.
5. When done, remove the loaf pan from the oven and let it rest for 5 minutes. Remove any fat that may have settled on the top.
6. Top with remaining cream cheese. Spread it all over. Sprinkle cheddar cheese and scallions.
7. Place the loaf pan back in the oven. Bake for 5 minutes.
8. Broil for 2-3 minutes or until the way you like the cheese to be browned.
9. Remove from the oven and let it rest for 5-10 minutes.

10. Slice and serve.

Breakfast BLT Salad

Serves: 4

Nutritional values per serving:

Calories – 292, Fat – 18 g, Carbohydrates – 18 g, Protein – 17.5 g

Ingredients:

- 6 cups Lacinato kale, discard hard stems and ribs, shredded
- 4 teaspoons extra virgin olive oil
- Black pepper to taste
- Salt to taste
- 4 large eggs
- 4 ounces avocado slices
- 2 teaspoons red wine vinegar
- 8 strips center cut bacon, cooked, chopped
- 20 grape tomatoes, halved

Method:

1. Place kale in a bowl. Drizzle olive oil and vinegar over it. Sprinkle salt.
2. Toss well. Massage the kale leaves using your hands for 3-4 minutes. It will soften.
3. Cook the eggs the way you desire.
4. Divide the kale among 4 serving bowls. Place bacon, tomatoes, avocado and egg on top of the kale in each bowl. Season with salt and pepper.
5. Serve.

Chocolate Waffles

Serves: 10

Nutritional values per serving:

Calories –289, Fat –26.6 g, Carbohydrates –7 g, Protein –7.2 g

Ingredients:

- 10 eggs
- 3 ½ tablespoons cocoa, unsweetened
- 2 teaspoon baking powder
- 6 tablespoons full fat milk or cream
- 3.8 ounces butter, melted
- 8 tablespoons coconut flour
- 8 tablespoons granulated sweetener of your choice
- 4 teaspoons vanilla extract

Method:

1. Crack the eggs and add whites into a large bowl. And yolks into another bowl.
2. Beat the whites until stiff peaks are formed.
3. Add coconut flour, baking powder, sweetener and baking powder into the bowl of yolks. Whisk well.
4. Add butter slowly and whisk simultaneously until smooth. Add vanilla and milk and whisk again.
5. Add this mixture into the bowl of whites and fold gently. Do not beat it; just fold lightly.
6. Preheat a waffle maker. Pour the batter into the waffle maker and cook until it is golden brown in color. Remove the waffles carefully and serve.
7. Repeat the above step with the remaining waffles.

Liver, Sausage and Eggs

Serves: 8

Nutritional values per serving:

Calories – 415, Fat – 19.3 g, Carbohydrates – 5.6 g, Protein – 52.6 g

Ingredients:

- 1 ½ pounds ground pork
- ½ pound ground beef liver
- 1 pound ground beef
- 1 teaspoon dried thyme
- 2 teaspoons dried sage
- 1 teaspoon dried rosemary
- 1 teaspoon pepper
- 1 teaspoon salt or to taste
- 8 large eggs
- 4 tablespoons olive oil

Method:

1. Add beef, pork, liver, salt, pepper and herbs into a bowl and mix well using your hands.
2. Divide the mixture into 8 equal portions and shape into patties. (You can also make into smaller size patties if desired)
3. Place a nonstick skillet over medium heat. Add a tablespoon of oil. Place 3-4 patties on it and cook until the patties are brown on both the sides and cooked inside.
4. Repeat the above step with the remaining patties.
5. Cook the eggs using the remaining oil as per your preference.
6. Serve patties with eggs.

Coconut Flour Porridge Breakfast Cereal

Serves: 2

Nutritional values per serving: Without toppings

Calories – 453, Fat – 39 g, Carbohydrates – 14 g, Protein – 13 g

Ingredients:

- 4 tablespoons coconut flour
- 1 ½ cups water
- 2 large eggs, beaten
- 2 tablespoons heavy cream or coconut milk
- 4 tablespoons golden flax meal
- A pinch last
- 4 teaspoons butter or ghee
- 2 tablespoons swerve or any other keto friendly sweetener

Method:

1. Add coconut flour, flax meal, water and salt into a heavy bottomed saucepan. Place the saucepan over medium heat.
2. Stir constantly. When it begins to bubble, lower heat and keep stirring until thick.
3. Turn off heat.
4. Add a little egg and whisk well. Repeat adding a little egg at the time until all of it is added, whisking each time.
5. Place the saucepan back over medium heat. Stir constantly until the porridge thickens further.
6. Turn off the heat and whisk for a minute. Add butter, cream and sweetener and whisk well.
7. Ladle into bowls and serve with toppings of your choice.

Chicken Kale Soup

Serves: 6

Nutritional values per serving:

Calories – 143, Fat – 2 g, Carbohydrates – 4 g, Protein – 23 g

Ingredients:

- 3 cups chicken breast, cooked, cubed
- 1 large onion, chopped
- 1 ½ tablespoons chicken bouillon granules or chicken broth mix
- A large pinch ground cloves
- Pepper to taste
- Salt to taste
- 18 ounces frozen kale
- 6 cups water or chicken broth
- ¾ teaspoon ground cinnamon
- 3 teaspoons garlic, minced

Method:

1. Place a soup pot over medium heat. Add all the ingredients into the pot. Bring to the boil.
2. Lower heat and simmer for 10-15 minutes. Taste and adjust the seasonings if necessary.
3. Ladle into soup bowls and serve.

Avgolemono (Greek Chicken Lemon and Egg Soup)

Serves: 4

Nutritional values per serving:

Calories – 289, Fat – 15 g, Carbohydrates – 4 g, Protein – 33 g

Ingredients:

- 2 cups cooked chicken, shredded
- 1 cup spaghetti squash, cooked
- 5 cups chicken broth or stock
- Salt to taste
- Pepper powder to taste
- 2-3 tablespoons fresh parsley, finely chopped
- Parmesan cheese, freshly grated (optional)

For the Avgolemono sauce:

- 2 medium eggs, at room temperature
- 1 ½-2 tablespoons lemon juice

Method:

1. Place the pot over medium heat. Add broth and bring to the boil.
2. Add chicken and spaghetti squash and heat thoroughly. Turn off the heat.
3. Meanwhile, make the Avgolemono sauce as follows: Beat the eggs until fluffy.
4. Add lemon juice and do not beat any more.
5. Add about a cup of the hot soup into the egg mixture whisking simultaneously.
6. Pour this into the pot and stir.
7. Add salt and pepper and stir.
8. Ladle into soup bowls and serve.

Creamy Garlic Chicken Soup

Serves: 6

Nutritional values per serving:

Calories – 307, Fat – 29 g, Carbohydrates – 2 g, Protein – 18 g

Ingredients:

- 3 tablespoons butter
- 6 ounces cream cheese, cubed
- 21 ounces chicken broth
- Salt to taste
- 3 cups cooked chicken breast, shredded
- 3 tablespoons Stacey Hawkins Garlic Gusto Seasoning
- 1/3 cup heavy cream

Method:

1. Place a saucepan over medium heat. Add butter. When butter melts, add chicken and mix until the chicken is well coated with the butter.
2. When the chicken is slightly heated, add cream cheese and seasoning and stir.
3. When cream cheese melts, add broth and cream and bring to the boil.
4. Lower heat and simmer uncovered for 5-6 minutes. Add salt and stir.
5. Ladle into soup bowls and serve.

Cream of Chicken Soup with Bacon

Serves: 6

Nutritional values per serving:

Calories – 247, Fat – 17.9 g, Carbohydrates – 5.3 g, Protein – 18.4 g

Ingredients:

- 9 slices bacon
- 3 cloves garlic, sliced
- 4 ½ cups chicken stock
- 6 ribs celery, chopped
- Salt to taste
- Pepper to taste
- 3 tablespoons butter
- 5 ounces shiitake mushrooms, sliced
- ¾ cup heavy cream
- 6 pieces cooked chicken thigh, skinless, boneless, chopped
- ¾ cup almond milk or coconut milk
- A handful fresh parsley chopped
- 2-3 tablespoons white wine or water

Method:

1. Place a soup pot over medium heat. Add 1 ½ of tablespoons butter. When the butter melts, add bacon and cook until crisp. Remove with a slotted spoon and place on a plate that is lined with paper towels.
2. Add remaining butter. When butter melts, add garlic and sauté for a couple of minutes until golden brown in color. Add mushrooms and sauté for 4-5 minutes.
3. Add water or wine and simmer until it reduces to half its original quantity.

4. Add chicken, celery, coconut milk, broth, cream salt and pepper. Stir well.
5. Ladle into soup bowls. Garnish with parsley and serve immediately.

Queso Soup

Serves: 3

Nutritional values per serving:

Calories – 332, Fat – 24.4 g, Carbohydrates – 7.1 g, Protein – 19 g

Ingredients:

- ½ pound ground beef
- 3 ounces cream cheese
- ¼ cup heavy whipping cream
- ½ packet taco seasoning
- ½ teaspoon garlic powder
- 1 small onion, chopped
- 1 can (10 ounces) diced tomatoes with green chilies
- 1 ¼ cups beef broth
- Salt to taste
- Pepper to taste

Method:

1. Place a soup pot over medium heat. Add beef and onions and cook until beef is brown. Break it simultaneously as it cooks.
2. Add cream cheese and mash it into the beef. Mix well.
3. Add cream, taco seasoning, beef broth, garlic powder and tomatoes and mix well.
4. Lower heat and simmer for 15-20 minutes. Season with salt and pepper.
5. Ladle into soup bowls and serve.

Kale and Sausage Soup

Serves: 9

Nutritional values per serving:

Calories – 298, Fat – 24 g, Carbohydrates – 8.49 g, Protein – 16 g

Ingredients:

- 1 ½ pounds ground sweet Italian sausage
- 1 large carrot, peeled, diced
- 1 large yellow onion, chopped
- ¾ medium head cauliflower, broken into florets
- 3 cloves garlic, crushed
- 4 ½ cups kale, discard hard stems and ribs, chopped
- 1 ½ tablespoons butter
- 3 tablespoons red wine vinegar
- 1 ½ teaspoons dried rubbed sage
- 1 ½ teaspoons dried oregano
- 1 teaspoon crushed red pepper flakes or to taste
- 1 ½ teaspoons dried basil
- 6 cups low sodium chicken broth
- Freshly ground pepper to taste
- Salt to taste
- 1 ½ cups heavy cream

Method:

1. Place a soup pot or a Dutch oven over medium high heat. Add sausage. Cook until brown. Break it simultaneously as it cooks.
2. Remove with a slotted spoon and place on a plate that is lined with a layer of paper towels.
3. Discard the fat left behind in the pot. Do not clean the pot though.

4. Place the pot back over medium heat.
5. Add onion and carrots and sauté until onions are translucent.
6. Add garlic and sauté until fragrant. Add vinegar and scrape the bottom of the pot to remove any brown bits that are stuck.
7. Add spices, herbs, stock and cream and bring to the boil.
8. Add cauliflower and lower the heat. Simmer without covering the pot until cauliflower is tender.
9. Add kale and the browned sausage. Mix well. Cook until kale wilts. Add salt and mix well.
10. Ladle into bowls and serve.

o Popper Soup

Nutritional values per serving:

Calories – 425, Fat – 38 g, Carbohydrates – 2.5 g, Protein – 17 g

Ingredients:

- 6 slices bacon
- ¾ cup heavy cream
- 3 tablespoons salsa Verde
- 1 ¼ cups Monterey Jack cheese, shredded
- 1 ¼ cups sharp cheddar cheese, shredded
- 6 large jalapeño peppers
- 6 ounces cream cheese
- 3 cups water or chicken broth
- 1 teaspoon garlic powder
- ½ teaspoon xanthan gum (optional)

Method:

1. Grill or broil the jalapeños until charred. Discard the skin and seeds and chop into fine pieces.
2. Meanwhile, place a soup pot over medium heat. Add bacon and cook until crisp. Remove with a slotted spoon and place on a plate that is lined with paper towels.
3. Do not discard the fat in the pot. Add cream, broth and cream cheese. Simmer until well combined.
4. Add jalapeños, salt pepper and xanthan gum if using and stir constantly until thick. Add both the cheeses and heat until cheese melts. Turn off the heat.
5. Ladle into soup bowls. Top with bacon and serve.

Creamy Mushroom, Fennel and Leek Soup

Serves: 6

Nutritional values per serving:

Calories – 708.7, Fat – 67 g, Carbohydrates – 17.5 g, Protein – 5.8 g

Ingredients:

- 6 cups vegetable stock, unsalted
- 13 ounces crimini mushrooms, sliced
- 1 ½ cups leeks, sliced
- 1 ½ cups fennel bulb, sliced, set aside some fronds, sliced
- 6 tablespoons butter, unsalted
- 4 ½ ounces dry sherry
- Salt to taste
- Pepper to taste
- 30 ounces heavy cream

Method:

1. Place a soup pot over high heat. Add stock and boil until it reduces to half its original quantity. Pour into a bowl and set aside.
2. Place the pot over medium heat. Add butter. When the butter melts, add mushrooms and sauté until light brown.
3. Add fennel and leeks and sauté until soft.
4. Add sherry. Scrape the bottom of the pot to remove any browned bits that may be stuck. Let it simmer for a while.
5. Add cream and allow it to boil.
6. Lower heat and stir constantly until it reduces to half its original quantity.

7. Add the stock that was set aside and stir. Remove from heat. Blend with an immersion blender until smooth.
8. Ladle into soup bowls. Garnish with fennel fronds and serve.

Broccoli Cheese Soup

Serves: 4

Nutritional values per serving:

Calories – 291, Fat – 25 g, Carbohydrates – 5 g, Protein – 13 g

Ingredients:

- 2 cups broccoli florets
- 1 ¾ cups chicken broth
- 1 ½ cups cheddar cheese, shredded
- 2 cloves garlic, minced
- ½ cup heavy cream
- Salt to taste
- Pepper to taste

Method:

1. Place a soup pot over medium heat. Add garlic and sauté for about a minute.
2. Add broth, broccoli and cream and bring to the boil.
3. Lower heat to low and simmer until broccoli is cooked. Add cheese and stir constantly until cheese melts.
4. Add salt and pepper and stir.
5. Ladle into soup bowls and serve.

Roasted Red Bell Pepper and Cauliflower Soup

Serves: 10

Nutritional values per serving:

Calories – 345, Fat – 32 g, Carbohydrates – 9 g, Protein – 6.4 g

Ingredients:

- ¾ cup duck fat, melted, divided
- 4 red bell peppers, halved, deseeded
- 6 green onions, sliced + extra to garnish
- 1 head cauliflower, chopped into florets
- 1 cup heavy cream
- 6 cups chicken broth
- 2 teaspoons garlic powder
- 2 teaspoons smoked paprika
- 2 teaspoons dried thyme + extra to garnish
- ½ teaspoon red pepper flakes
- Salt to taste
- Pepper to taste
- 8 ounces goats cheese, crumbled, to garnish

Method:

1. Place the peppers in a preheated oven and broil for 10-15 minutes or until the skin gets slightly charred. Transfer into a container with a lid. Close lid and set aside for a while. Uncover and peel the skin of the peppers.
2. Place the cauliflower on a baking sheet. Drizzle 4 tablespoons duck fat, salt and pepper over the cauliflower and bake at 400° F for about 30 minutes or until roasted.

3. Place a soup pot over medium heat. Add remaining duck fat and green onions. Sauté for a couple of minutes.
4. Add peppers, spices, broth and salt and simmer for 15-20 minutes.
5. Blend with an immersion blender until smooth.
6. Add cream and mix well.
7. Ladle into soup bowls. Top with goat's cheese. Sprinkle thyme and green onions and serve. Garnish with some crispy bacon and serve.

Creamy Red Gazpacho

Serves: 3

Nutritional values per serving:

Calories – 528, Fat – 50.8 g, Carbohydrates – 14.3 g, Protein – 7.5 g

Ingredients:

- 1 small red bell pepper, halved
- 1 small green bell pepper, halved
- 1 small red onion, chopped
- 2-3 medium tomatoes, quartered, deseeded
- 1 medium avocado, peeled, pitted, chopped
- 1 clove garlic, peeled
- 1 medium spring onion, thinly sliced
- 1 tablespoon apple cider vinegar
- 1 medium cucumber, finely chopped
- ½ teaspoon salt or to taste
- ½ cup extra virgin olive oil + extra to drizzle
- Freshly ground pepper to taste
- 3.5 ounces soft goat's cheese, crumbled
- 1 tablespoon lemon juice
- 2 tablespoons basil leaves, chopped+ extra to garnish
- 2 tablespoons parsley, chopped + extra to garnish

Method:

1. Place the pepper halves on a lined baking sheet with the cut side facing down.
2. Roast in a preheated oven at 400° F for about 20 minutes or until roasted and charred. Remove from the oven and cool. Peel and discard the skin.
3. Add onion, avocado, roasted peppers, parsley, basil, garlic, oil, vinegar, salt and pepper into a blender and blend until smooth.

4. Pour into a bowl. Add cucumber and spring onion and stir. Add salt and pepper to taste. Mix well.
5. Ladle into bowls. Sprinkle goat's cheese, parsley and basil on top and serve.
6. Serve at room temperature or chilled.

Chapter Seven: Ketogenic Smoothie Recipes

Strawberry & Rhubarb Pie Smoothie

Serves: 2

Nutritional values per serving:

Calories – 392, Fat – 31.8 g, Carbohydrates – 14.7 g, Protein – 14.2 g

Ingredients:

- 8 strawberries
- 2 large eggs
- 4 medium rhubarb stalks
- 1 cup almond milk
- 2 ounces almonds or 4 tablespoons almond butter
- 4 tablespoons full fat cream or coconut milk
- 1 teaspoon pure vanilla bean extract
- 2 teaspoons fresh ginger root, grated
- 10-12 drops liquid stevia or to taste

Method:

1. Add strawberries, eggs, rhubarb stalks, almond milk, almonds, cream, vanilla extract, ginger and stevia into a blender until smooth.
2. Pour into tall glasses and serve with crushed ice.

Fat Bomb Chocolate Smoothie

Serves: 2

Nutritional values per serving:

Calories – 570, Fat – 46 g, Carbohydrates – 6.2 g, Protein – 34.5 g

Ingredients:

- 4 large eggs or 4 tablespoons chia seeds or 4 tablespoons almond butter or 4 tablespoons coconut butter
- ½ cup chocolate or plain whey protein powder or egg white protein powder or collagen powder
- ½ cup heavy whipping cream or coconut milk
- 2 tablespoons MCT oil or extra virgin coconut oil
- 6-8 drops stevia extract
- 1 teaspoon ground cinnamon or vanilla extract (optional)
- 2 tablespoons cacao powder, unsweetened
- ½ cup water
- 1 cup ice cubes

Method:

1. Add all the ingredients into a blender and blend until smooth.
2. Pour into tall glasses and serve.

Healthy Keto Green Smoothie

Serves: 2

Nutritional values per serving:

Calories – 11.4, Fat – 48.2 g, Carbohydrates – 11.4 g, Protein – 4.2 g

Ingredients:

- 1 medium avocado, peeled, pitted, chopped
- 1 cup coconut milk or ½ cup heavy whipping cream along with ½ cup water
- 1 teaspoon vanilla powder or vanilla extract
- 4 tablespoons stevia or stevia drops to taste
- 1 cup fresh spinach
- 1-1 ½ cups water
- Ice cubes, as required
- 2 tablespoons MCT oil or extra virgin coconut oil
- 2 teaspoons matcha powder (optional)

Method:

1. Add all the ingredients into a blender and blend until smooth.
2. Pour into tall glasses and serve.

Healthy Green Shake

Serves: 2

Nutritional values per serving:

Calories – 380, Fat – 30 g, Carbohydrates – 13 g, Protein – 12 g

Ingredients:

- 4 cups spinach or kale
- 4 Brazil nuts
- 2 scoops Amazing Grass Greens powder
- 2 cups coconut milk
- 2 tablespoons psyllium seeds or husk (optional)
- 20 almonds
- 2 scoops whey protein powder (optional)

Method:

1. Add spinach, Brazil nuts, almonds and coconut milk into a blender and blend until smooth.
2. Add spinach, greens powder, psyllium seeds or husk and protein powder.
3. Blend until smooth.
4. Pour into tall glasses and serve with crushed ice.

Green Lemon Smoothie

Serves: 2

Nutritional values per serving:

Calories – 339, Fat – 22.6 g, Carbohydrate – 12.7 g, Protein – 21.5 g

Ingredients:

- 1 large avocado, peeled, pitted, chopped
- 6 tablespoons lemon juice
- 1 cup coconut milk or coconut cream
- 2 scoops bulletproof collagen protein
- 2 cups ice cubes
- 1 cucumber, chopped
- 4 cups fresh spinach, chopped
- 2 tablespoons brain octane oil
- 2 scoops bulletproof whey protein
- Stevia to taste
- 5-6 drops lemon essential oil

Method:

1. Lightly steam the spinach leaves in the steaming equipment you have. Cool completely.
2. Add all the ingredients into a blender and blend until smooth.
3. Pour into tall glasses and serve.

Strawberry Almond Smoothie

Serves: 1

Nutritional values per serving:

Calories – 304, Fat – 25 g, Carbohydrates – 7 g, Protein – 15 g

Ingredients:

- 8 ounces almond milk, unsweetened
- 2 ounces heavy cream
- ½ scoop whey vanilla Isolate powder
- Stevia to taste
- 1/8 cup frozen strawberries, unsweetened

Method:

1. Add almond milk, cream, whey protein, stevia and strawberries into a blender and blend until smooth.
2. Pour into a tall glass and serve.

Coco-Nut Milkshake

Serves: 2

Nutritional values per serving:

Calories – 79.l, Fat – 5.7 g, Carbohydrate – 6.4 g, Protein – 3.6 g

Ingredients:

- 2 cups coconut milk
- 2 tablespoons natural peanut butter, unsweetened
- A pinch sea salt
- 2 tablespoons cocoa powder, unsweetened
- 10 drops stevia or to taste

Method:

1. Add coconut milk, peanut butter, salt, cocoa powder and stevia into a blender and blend until smooth and frothy.
2. Pour into glasses and serve with crushed ice.

Orange Creamsicle Cooler

Serves: 1

Nutritional values per serving:

Calories −290, Fat − 25 g, Carbohydrates − 4 g, Protein − 15 g

Ingredients:

- 8 ounces almond milk, unsweetened
- 2 ounces heavy cream
- ½ scoop Jay Robb Tropical Dreamsicle whey protein powder
- Stevia to taste

Method:

1. Add almond milk, cream, whey protein and stevia into a blender and blend until smooth.
2. Pour into a tall glass and serve.

Raspberry Avocado Smoothie

Serves: 1

Nutritional values per serving:

Calories – 227, Fat – 20 g, Carbohydrates – 12.8 g, Protein – 2.5 g

Ingredients:

- ½ ripe avocado, peeled, pitted, chopped
- 1 ½ tablespoons lemon juice
- ¼ cup frozen raspberries, unsweetened
- 2/3 cup water
- 1 tablespoon Stevia or any other sugar substitute

Method:

1. Add all the ingredients into a blender and blend until smooth.
2. Pour into tall glasses and serve.

Blackberry Cheesecake Smoothie

Serves: 2

Nutritional values per serving:

Calories – 515, Fat – 53 g, Carbohydrates – 10.8 g, Protein – 6.4 g

Ingredients:

- 1 cup blackberries, fresh or frozen
- ½ cup heavy whipping cream or coconut milk
- 2 tablespoons MCT oil or extra virgin coconut oil
- 6-8 drops stevia or to taste
- ½ cup full fat cream cheese or creamed coconut milk
- 1 cup water
- 1 teaspoon sugar free vanilla extract or ½ teaspoon pure vanilla powder

Method:

1. Add blackberries, cream MCT oil, stevia, cream cheese, water and vanilla into a blender and blend until smooth.
2. Pour into tall glasses and serve.

Low Carb Smoothie Bowl

Serves: 2

Nutritional values per serving:

Calories – 570, Fat – 25 g, Carbohydrates – 4 g, Protein – 35 g

Ingredients:

For smoothie bowl base:

- 2 cups spinach
- 4 tablespoons heavy cream
- 2 scoops whey protein powder or any other low carb protein powder
- 2 tablespoons coconut oil
- 4 ice cubes
- 1 cup almond milk

For toppings:

- 8 raspberries
- 2 tablespoons shredded coconut, unsweetened
- 8 walnuts, chopped
- 2 teaspoons chia seeds

Method:

1. Add spinach into the blender. Add almond milk, coconut oil, cream and ice.
2. Blend until smooth.
3. Divide equally and pour into 2 bowls.
4. Add toppings and serve.

Chapter Eight: Ketogenic Salad Recipes

Crunchy and Nutty Cauliflower Salad

Serves: 6

Nutritional values per serving:

Calories −160, Fat − 14.3 g, Net Carbohydrates − 3.8 g, Protein − 4.1 g

Ingredients:

- 6 cups cauliflower, finely chopped
- 1 cup walnuts, chopped
- 2 cups leeks, green parts only, finely chopped
- Sea salt to taste
- 2 cups sour cream

Method:

1. Add all the ingredients into an airtight container. Toss well. Close the lid.
2. Chill for 3-4 hours for the flavors to set in.
3. Serve.

Mediterranean Chopped Salad

Serves: 2

Nutritional values per serving:

Calories – 113, Fat – 10 g, Carbohydrates – 5 g, Protein – 1 g

Ingredients:

- 1 medium tomato, deseeded, chopped
- 2 scallions, chopped
- 2 tablespoons Kalamata olives pitted, coarsely chopped
- 1 small seedless cucumber, chopped
- A handful fresh parsley, chopped
- 1 tablespoon extra-virgin olive oil
- Salt to taste
- ½ tablespoon white wine vinegar
- Freshly ground pepper to taste

Method:

1. Add all the ingredients into a bowl and toss well.
2. Serve right away.

Mock Potato Salad

Serves: 4

Nutritional values per serving:

Calories – 254, Fat – 21.1 g, Carbohydrates – 10.5 g, Protein – 6.6 g

Ingredients:

For salad:

- 3 large eggs, hard boiled, peeled, chopped into bite sized pieces
- 1 small turnip, peeled, chopped into ½ inch pieces
- 1 small celeriac, peeled, chopped into ½ inch pieces
- 1 small rutabaga, chopped into ½ inch pieces
- 1 small onion, finely chopped
- 2-3 pickled cucumber, diced
- 1 medium stalk celery, sliced

For dressing:

- ½ teaspoon Dijon mustard
- 6 tablespoons Keto friendly mayonnaise
- 1 tablespoon pickle juice or vinegar
- ½ teaspoon celery seeds
- 1 tablespoon chives, chopped
- A handful fresh parsley, chopped
- Salt to taste
- Freshly ground pepper to taste

Spices to boil vegetables:

- 1 bay leaf
- ½ teaspoons black peppercorns
- ½ tablespoon apple cider vinegar
- 1 teaspoon salt

Method:

1. Place a pot of water over high heat. Add vinegar, peppercorns, salt, and bay leaves.
2. Add rutabaga, turnips and celeriac and bring to the boil.
3. Lower heat and simmer until vegetables are tender. Discard the spices and drain water.
4. Transfer the cooked vegetables into a bowl and let it cool.
5. Add rest of the ingredients of salad into it and toss well.
6. Add all the ingredients of the dressing into a bowl and mix well.
7. Pour dressing over the salad. Toss well. Taste and adjust the seasoning to taste.

Chicken Salad Picnic Eggs

Serves: 4

Nutritional values per serving:

Calories −288, Fat − 16 g, Carbohydrates − 1 g, Protein − NA

Ingredients:

- 12 eggs, hard boiled, peeled, halved lengthwise
- 4 tablespoons keto friendly mayonnaise
- 1 small onion, chopped
- 1 teaspoon dill
- Old bay seasoning to taste
- 2 cups chicken, cooked, finely chopped
- 2 teaspoons Dijon mustard
- ¼ teaspoon celery salt
- 1 teaspoon lemon pepper seasoning

Method:

1. Scoop out the yolk from the eggs and add into a bowl. Set the whites aside.
2. Add rest of the ingredients except old bay seasoning to the bowl of yolks. Mix well.
3. Refrigerate for a while.
4. Stuff this mixture in the egg whites. Place some on top too.
5. Sprinkle old bay seasoning on top and serve.

Tuna Salad

Serves: 4

Nutritional values per serving: ½ cup

Calories – 248, Fat – 19 g, Carbohydrates – 2 g, Protein – 20 g

Ingredients:

- 4 cans tuna (2 cups), drained
- 2 teaspoons dried onion flakes
- 6 tablespoons keto friendly mayonnaise
- Salt to taste
- Pepper to taste

Method:

1. Add tuna, onion flakes and mayonnaise into a bowl and toss well.
2. Sprinkle salt and pepper and toss again.
3. Serve.

Chicken Cobb Salad

Serves: 2

Nutritional values per serving:

Calories – 504, Fat – 30.3 g, Carbohydrates – 10.2 g, Protein – 47.1 g

Ingredients:

- 1 chicken breast, skinless, boneless, cooked, sliced
- 2 hard boiled eggs, peeled, sliced or chopped
- 1 avocado, peeled, pitted, chopped
- 4 tablespoons blue cheese dressing (optional)
- 4 cups spring mix
- 4 slices thick cut bacon, cooked until crisp, chopped
- 2 ounces blue cheese, crumbled
- 8 grape tomatoes

Method:

1. Divide the spring mix into 2 bowls or plates.
2. Divide and place chicken, egg, bacon, avocado and blue cheese on it.
3. Top with tomatoes and blue cheese dressing.
4. Serve right away.

Lemon Blueberry Chicken Salad

Serves: 2

Nutritional values per serving: 1 large bowl

Calories – 490, Fat – 42 g, Carbohydrates – 5 g, Protein – 27 g

Ingredients:

- 20 blueberries
- 2 large bags salad leaves (about 4.5 ounces each)
- 4 teaspoons fresh lemon juice
- 4 tablespoons coconut oil
- 1 small onion, sliced
- 4 tablespoons olive oil
- 1 pound chicken breast, boneless, skinless, chopped into bite size pieces
- Salt to taste
- Pepper to taste

Method:

1. Place a skillet over medium heat. Add coconut oil. When oil melts, add chicken and cook until done.
2. Add salt and pepper and sauté for a minute.
3. Transfer into a serving bowl. Add blueberries, onion, olive oil, salad leaves and lemon juice and toss well.
4. Divide into individual serving bowls and serve.

Curried Chicken Salad

Serves: 4

Nutritional values per serving:

Calories – 385, Fat – 30 g, Carbohydrates – 7 g, Protein – 23 g

Ingredients:

- 2 chicken breasts, skinless, boneless, cut into small pieces
- 1 red bell pepper, chopped
- 1 medium onion, chopped
- Coconut oil, as required
- 1 zucchini or cucumber, cubed
- 28-30 blueberries
- 2 tablespoons curry powder
- 4 tablespoons fresh cilantro, finely chopped
- Lettuce leaves to serve
- 2 tablespoons pumpkin seeds
- ½ cup coconut cream
- Salt to taste

Method:

1. Place a skillet over medium heat. Add a teaspoon of coconut oil. Add onions and sauté until translucent. Transfer into a serving bowl.
2. Place the skillet back over heat. Add 2-3 tablespoons coconut oil. When the oil is melted, add chicken and cook until tender.
3. Transfer into the bowl of onions. Let the chicken cool.
4. Add bell pepper, blueberries, zucchini or cucumber and pumpkin seeds and toss well.
5. Add curry powder, coconut cream, cilantro and salt and toss well.

6. Serve over lettuce leaves.

Easy Russian Slaw

Serves: 3

Nutritional values per serving:

Calories – 131, Fat – 11.1 g, Carbohydrates – 8.3 g, Protein – 1.7 g

Ingredients:

- 2.5 ounces red cabbage, thinly sliced
- 4.4 ounces green or white cabbage, thinly sliced
- 2 ounces fennel bulb, thinly sliced
- 1.4 ounces celeriac, grated

For Russian dressing:

- 3 tablespoon mayonnaise
- ½ tablespoon Sriracha chili sauce
- ½ teaspoon horseradish, freshly grated
- 1 tablespoon fresh parsley, finely chopped
- 1 tablespoon lemon juice
- 1 tablespoon chives, finely chopped
- 1 small pickled cucumber
- 1 tablespoon sour cream or coconut milk
- Freshly ground pepper to taste
- Salt to taste

Method:

1. Add all the ingredients of dressing into a bowl and mix well.
2. Add all the vegetables into a bowl and toss well. Pour dressing on top. Fold gently and serve.

Grilled Vegetable Salad with Olive oil and Feta

Serves: 2

Nutritional values per serving:

Calories – 186, Fat – 14 g, Carbohydrates – 12 g, Protein – 5 g

Ingredients:

- 1 small eggplant, cut into ¼ inch thick slices
- 1 small red bell pepper, cut into ½ inch strips
- 1 small zucchini, cut into ¼ inch thick slices
- 1 ½ tablespoons extra-virgin olive oil
- Salt to taste
- 1 clove garlic, minced
- Freshly cracked pepper to taste
- ¼ cup feta cheese, crumbled
- ¼ teaspoon dried oregano

Method:

1. Place the vegetables on a preheated grill and grill until the vegetables are slightly charred on the edges. Turn the vegetables and grill for 2-3 minutes more.
2. Cool the vegetables and cut into smaller pieces. Add into a bowl.
3. Add rest of the ingredients and toss until well combined.
4. Serve.

Chapter Nine: Ketogenic Snack Recipes

Rainbow Goat's Cheese Balls

Serves: 10

Nutritional values per serving: 1 ball

Calories – 59, Fat – 5 g, Carbohydrates – 0 g, Protein – 3 g

Ingredients:

- 5.5 ounces soft goat's cheese, rind less
- Salt to taste
- 1-2 teaspoons extra virgin olive oil
-

For covering:

- 2-3 teaspoon white sesame seeds, toasted
- 2-3 teaspoon black sesame seeds, toasted
- Snipped chives to taste
- Pink peppercorns, crushed to taste
- Cayenne pepper to taste
-

Method:

1. Add goat's cheese and oil into a bowl. Mash well.
2. Add salt and mix well.
3. Divide the mixture into 10 equal portions and shape into balls.
4. Dredge the balls in all the covering ingredients.
5. Serve.

Italian Style Zucchini Rolls

Serves: 8 (7 rolls per serving)

Nutritional values per serving:

Calories – 257, Fat – 19.2 g, Carbohydrates – 6.3 g, Protein – 15.7 g

Ingredients:

- 6 small or baby zucchinis
- 2 cups soft goat's cheese
- ½ cup raspberry vinegar or any other fruit vinegar
- 28 thin slices streaky bacon
- 1 cup sun dried tomatoes, drained, chopped
- 1 cup fresh basil, chopped

Method:

1. Use a peeler and make thin strips of the zucchinis.
2. Add vinegar into a bowl. Add zucchini strips into the bowl. The strips should dip into the vinegar. Set aside for about 10 minutes.
3. Meanwhile line a baking sheet with parchment paper. Place bacon strips on the baking sheet.
4. Bake in a preheated oven at 400° F for 5 minutes or until slightly crisp.
5. Remove from the oven.
6. Lay the zucchini strips on your work area. Place a strip of bacon on each zucchini strip. Sprinkle cheese on it. Place a piece of tomato and sprinkle basil on it. Roll each set. Insert a toothpick in each.
7. Serve.

Bacon-Goat Cheese Jalapeno Poppers

Serves: 4

Nutritional values per serving: 2 pepper halves

Calories – 59, Fat – 3.9 g, Carbohydrates – 3 g, Protein – 3 g

Ingredients:

- 4 ounces goat's cheese, softened
- 2 teaspoons red onion, grated
- Pepper to taste
- Kosher salt to taste
- A large pinch garlic powder
- 1 ounce 1/3 less fat cream cheese, softened
- 4 medium jalapeño peppers, halved lengthwise, deseeded
- 1 tablespoon red pepper jelly
- 1 ½ center – cup bacon slices, cooked, crumbled
- A few drops water if required

Method:

1. Add goat's cheese, cream cheese, onion, salt, pepper and garlic powder into a bowl and mix well.
2. Place the bell peppers on a rimmed baking sheet.
3. Fill the bell peppers with the cheese mixture.
4. Broil in a preheated oven for 7 minutes. Sprinkle bacon on top.
5. Add red pepper jelly into a small microwave safe bowl. Add 20-30 drops water in it.
6. Microwave on high for 20-25 seconds or until melted. Stir and pour over the peppers. Serve right away.

Marinated Olives and Feta

Serves: 6

Nutritional values per serving: 2 tablespoons

Calories – 73, Fat – 7 g, Carbohydrates – 2 g, Protein – 1 g

Ingredients:

- ½ cup Kalamata or mixed Greek olives, pitted, sliced
- 1 tablespoon extra-virgin olive oil
- ¼ cup low fat feta cheese, chopped
- 1 teaspoon fresh rosemary, chopped
- Freshly ground black pepper to taste
- A pinch crushed red pepper
- Zest of ½ lemon
- Juice of ½ lemon
- 1 clove garlic, thinly sliced
- Salt to taste

Method:

1. Add all the ingredients to a bowl and toss well.
2. Set aside for a while for the flavors to set in.
3. Toss and serve.

Fish Fingers

Serves: 6

Nutritional values per serving: Without dip

Calories – 422, Fat – 26 g, Carbohydrates – 12 g, Protein – 33 g

Ingredients:

- 6 ounces white fish, rinsed, cut into fingers
- ½ teaspoon garlic powder
- 1 egg, beaten
- 2 tablespoons coconut flour
- 1 tablespoons seasoned salt or to taste
- 1 teaspoon garlic powder
- Pepper powder to taste
- ½ cup coconut oil

Method:

1. Add coconut flour, seasoned salt, garlic powder and pepper powder into a bowl.
2. First dip the fish fingers in the egg and then roll in the coconut mixture and set aside on a plate.
3. Add ¼ cup oil to a small, deep pan and place over medium heat.
4. Fry the fish fingers in batches until brown.
5. Serve with any keto friendly dip of your choice.

Low Carb Pizza Bites

Serves: 6

Nutritional values per serving:

Calories – 102, Fat – 7 g, Carbohydrates – 1.3 g, Protein – 8.6 g

Ingredients:

- 5.5 ounces mozzarella cheese, grated
- Few slices salami or Parma ham, cut into small pieces
- 6 teaspoons Keto friendly marinara sauce
- Handful basil leaves, chopped

Method:

1. Take a baking sheet and place small mounds (1-2 tablespoons) of mozzarella cheese on it. Leave sufficient gap between 2 mounds. In all there should be either 6 bigger mounds or 12 smaller mounds)
2. Broil in a preheated oven until top is brown. The cheese will melt and spread so the gaps between 2 mounds are necessary. Remove from the oven and set aside to cool. It will harden in a while. This is the pizza base.
3. Meanwhile, place a skillet over medium heat. Add salami and cook until brown.
4. Place the pizza bases on a serving platter. Spread a teaspoon of marinara sauce over each.
5. Place salami pieces on each. Sprinkle basil on top and serve.

Spicy Chicken Nuggets

Serves: 2

Nutritional values per serving:

Calories – 360, Fat – 11.5 g, Carbohydrates – 1.5 g, Protein – 61.5 g

Ingredients:

- 16 ounces chicken tenders, chop into bite sized pieces
- 1 ounce pork rinds
- Salt to taste
- Pepper powder to taste
- 2 tablespoons almond flour
- 1 egg, beaten
- ¼ teaspoon chili powder
- Cayenne pepper to taste
- ¼ teaspoon garlic powder
- ½ teaspoon onion powder
- ¼ teaspoon Creole seasoning

Method:

1. Blend together pork rind, onion and garlic powder, Creole seasoning, almond flour, salt, pepper, chili powder and cayenne pepper in a blender. Transfer into a bowl.
2. First dip a chicken nugget in egg. Shake to drop off excess egg and then dredge in the almond flour mixture. Place on a greased baking sheet.
3. Repeat with the remaining nuggets.
4. Bake in a preheated oven at 400° F for 20 minutes or until brown and crisp.

Mini Cheese Balls

Serves: 9

Nutritional values per serving: 2 balls

Calories – 94, Fat – 7.4 g, Carbohydrates – 2 g, Protein – 5 g

Ingredients:

- 4 ounces plain almond milk cream cheese
- 4 ounces goat's cheese
- ¼ teaspoon lemon zest, grated
- A handful fresh thyme, finely chopped
- ¼ cup roasted, salted almonds, chopped

Method:

1. Add goat's cheese, cream cheese and lemon zest in a bowl.
2. Beat with an electric mixer on medium speed until smooth. Place the bowl in the freezer for 15 minutes.
3. Add nuts and thyme into the food processor bowl and pulse until fine. Transfer into a bowl.
4. Divide the mixture into 18 equal portions and shape into balls.
5. Dredge the balls in the nut mixture. Cover and chill until use.

Smoked Paprika Zucchini Chips

Serves: 7-8

Nutritional values per serving: 20 chips

Calories – 35, Fat – 3 g, Carbohydrates – 2 g, Protein – 0.6 g

Ingredients:

- 3 medium zucchinis
- Salt to taste
- Olive oil cooking spray
- 3 -4 teaspoons smoked paprika
- 2 teaspoons onion powder
- Pepper powder to taste

Method:

1. Cut the zucchini into 1/8th inch thick slices, crosswise with a mandolin slicer or a sharp knife.
2. Place the zucchini on a sieve in layers sprinkled with salt and pepper. Keep aside for an hour. Some moisture content of the zucchini will drain out.
3. Pat dry the zucchini slices with a paper towel and place on a greased baking tray.
4. Brush the top of the slices with oil. Sprinkle onion powder, paprika and pepper.
5. Bake in a preheated oven at 250° F for 45 minutes. Rotate the baking tray 2-3 times while baking.
6. Turn off the oven and let the chips remain inside for an hour so that it remains crispy.
7. Transfer into an airtight container.

Zucchini Pizza Bites

Serves: 5

Nutritional values per serving: 2 bites

Calories – 117, Fat – 8 g, Carbohydrates – 4 g, Protein – 8 g

Ingredients:

- 1 medium zucchini, shredded
- 1 tablespoon coconut flour
- Pepper to taste
- Salt to taste
- ½ tablespoon butter, melted
- 2/3 cups mozzarella cheese, shredded
- 1 large egg

For topping:

- 2 tablespoons marinara sauce
- ½ teaspoon Italian seasoning
- 2/3 cup mozzarella cheese, shredded + extra to garnish
- ½ ounce pepperoni mini slices or regular slices, quartered

Method:

1. Place silicone liners or parchment papers liners in 10 cups of mini muffin pan.
2. Add zucchini, mozzarella, and coconut flour into a bowl and mix well. Add butter, egg, salt and pepper and mix well.
3. Divide the mixture into the prepared muffin cups. Spread the mixture evenly and the top is smooth.
4. Bake in a preheated oven at 375° F for 18-22 minutes or until the top set and golden brown in color.

5. Remove from the oven and cool for a while. Spread a teaspoon of marinara sauce over each bite.
6. Sprinkle mozzarella cheese and Italian seasoning. Place pepperoni slices on top.
7. Broil for a couple of minutes until the cheese melts and serve.

Cucumber Bites

Serves: 2

Nutritional values per serving:

Calories – 140, Fat – 10 g, Net Carbohydrates – 3 g, Protein – 7 g

Ingredients:

- 1 medium cucumber, cut into ¼ inch thick round slices
- 2 ounces smoked salmon, cut into pieces
- ½ small avocado, peeled, pitted, cut into small slices
- 1 teaspoon black sesame seeds

Method:

1. Place cucumber slices on a serving platter. Place avocado slices over it.
2. Place salmon over it. Sprinkle sesame seeds on top and serve.

Avocado Balls

Serves: 12

Nutritional values per serving:

Calories – 156, Fat – 15.2 g, Carbohydrate – 2.7 g, Protein – 3.4 g

Ingredients:

- 1 large avocado, peeled, pitted, chopped
- 4 cloves garlic, crushed
- 1 small white onion, chopped
- Freshly ground black or cayenne pepper
- ¼ cup fresh cilantro, chopped
- ½ cup ghee or butter, at room temperature
- 2 small chili peppers, finely chopped
- 2 tablespoons fresh lime juice
- ½ teaspoon salt or to taste
- 8 large slices bacon

Method:

1. Place a nonstick pan over medium heat. Add bacon and cook until crisp.
2. Remove with a slotted spoon and place on a place that is lined with paper towels. When cool enough to handle, crumble and set aside. Retain the bacon fat.
3. Add all the ingredients except onions into a bowl. Mash well.
4. Add onion and mix until well combined. Add the retained bacon fat and mix again.
5. Cover and chill for 30-40 minutes.

6. Divide the mixture into 12 equal portions and shape into balls.
7. Dredge the balls in crumbled bacon and place on a serving platter. Refrigerate for a while and serve.

Pesto Keto Crackers

Serves: 12

Nutritional values per serving:

Calories –210, Fat –20 g, Carbohydrates –5.5 g, Protein –5 g

Ingredients:

<u>Dry ingredients:</u>

- 2 ½ cups almond flour
- 1 teaspoon salt
- ½ teaspoon dried basil
- ½ teaspoon ground black pepper
- 1 teaspoon baking powder
- ½ teaspoon cayenne pepper or to taste

<u>Wet ingredients:</u>

- 2 cloves garlic, peeled, pressed
- 6 tablespoons butter, chopped into small pieces
- 4 tablespoons basil pesto

Method:

1. Place a sheet of parchment paper on a large baking sheet. Set aside. Use 2 baking sheets if required.
2. Mix together all the dry ingredients in a large bowl.
3. Add basil and mix well using your hands until coarse crumbs are formed.
4. Add butter and mix with your hands until dough is formed.
5. Spread the dough on the prepared baking sheet evenly such that it is about 1 ½ mm in thickness. Use 2 baking sheets if required.
6. Bake in a preheated oven at 325°F for about 15 minutes until light golden brown.

7. Remove the baking sheet from the oven and chop into 12 equal crackers or into smaller crackers if desired. Cool completely.
8. Transfer into an airtight container at room temperature. It can last for a week.

Chapter Ten: Ketogenic Side Dish Recipes

Cauliflower Cheese & Onion Croquettes

Serves: 2 (makes 6 croquettes)

Nutritional values per serving: 1 croquette

Calories – 86, Fat – 6 g, Carbohydrates – 2.6 g, Protein – 5 g

Ingredients:

- 1 small cauliflower, chopped into florets
- 1 teaspoon garlic powder
- ¼ cup cheddar cheese, grated
- ¼ teaspoon salt
- 1 tablespoon olive oil
- ½ cup Parmesan cheese, grated
- 2 spring onions, finely chopped
- ¼ teaspoon Dijon mustard
- ¼ teaspoon pepper

Method:

1. Place a saucepan over medium heat. Add cauliflower and cover with water. When it begins to boil, lower heat and cover with a lid.
2. Simmer until tender. Drain and squeeze out excess water from the cauliflower.
3. Add cauliflower into a bowl and mash well.
4. Add spring onions, cheddar cheese, Parmesan cheese, mustard, garlic powder, salt and pepper. Mix well.
5. Divide the mixture into 6 equal portions and shape into croquettes.

6. Place a sheet of parchment paper on a plate. Place croquettes on it. Chill for 30-40 minutes.
7. Place a nonstick pan over medium heat. Add oil. When the oil is heated, place croquettes and cook until golden brown. Flip sides and cook the other side too.
8. Cook in batches if required.

Cheese and Jalapeño Bread

Serves: 8 slices

Nutritional values per serving:

Calories −137, Fat −11 g, Carbohydrates −4 g, Protein −6 g

Ingredients:

Wet ingredients:

- 8 eggs
- ½ cup water
- ½ cup butter

Dry ingredients:

- 2/3 cup coconut flour
- 1 teaspoon garlic powder
- ½ teaspoon baking powder
- 1 teaspoon pepper powder
- 1 teaspoon salt

Other ingredients:

- 1 cup cheddar cheese, grated
- ½ cup Parmesan cheese, grated
- 8 jalapeño chilies, deseeded, chopped

Method:

1. Grease a loaf pan with a little butter or olive oil. Line it with parchment paper. Set aside.
2. Add all the dry ingredients into a bowl. Mix well.
3. Add all the wet ingredients into a large bowl. Whisk until well combined.
4. Add the dry ingredients into the bowl of wet ingredients and whisk until well combined.
5. Add jalapeños, cheddar cheese and Parmesan cheese and fold gently.

6. Pour into the prepared loaf pan.
7. Bake in a preheated oven at 400° F for about 20-25 minutes or until light brown on top and on the edges.
8. Cut into 8 equal slices and serve.

Cheesy Cauliflower Gratin

Serves: 3

Nutritional values per serving:

Calories – 215, Fat – 19 g, Net Carbohydrates – 2 g, Protein – 6 g

Ingredients:

- 2 cups cauliflower florets
- 3 tablespoons heavy whipping cream
- 3 deli slices pepper Jack cheese
- 2 tablespoons butter
- Salt to taste
- Pepper to taste

Method:

1. Add cauliflower, cream, butter, salt and pepper into a microwave safe dish.
2. Microwave on High for 15-20 minutes or until soft. Check the cauliflower after 10 minutes and after that every 2-3 minutes.
3. When done, mash with a fork.
4. Taste and adjust the seasoning if necessary.
5. Place cheese slices on top. Microwave on High for a couple of minutes until cheese melts.
6. Serve right away.

Colcannon

Serves: 2

Nutritional values per serving:

Calories – 112, Fat – 5 g, Carbohydrates – 16 g, Protein – 6 g

Ingredients:

- 3 cups cauliflower florets
- 1 ½ cups kale, discard hard stems and ribs
- 3 tablespoons fat free milk
- 2 teaspoons butter
- Freshly ground pepper to taste
- 1 teaspoon salt
- 1 scallion, chopped
- 2 cloves garlic, crushed

Method:

1. Add cauliflower into a microwave safe bowl and cover with a lid. Microwave on high for 10-15 minutes until tender
2. Place a pan over medium heat. Add ½ teaspoon butter. When butter melts, add garlic and scallions and sauté until fragrant.
3. Add kale and salt and cook until it wilts. Turn off the heat. Transfer into a serving bowl.
4. Add cauliflower into a blender. Add milk and blend until smooth.
5. Transfer into the serving bowl. Add 1-teaspoon butter, salt and pepper and stir.
6. Top with remaining ½ teaspoon butter and serve immediately.

Loaded Mashed Cheesy Pancetta Cauliflower

Serves: 6

Nutritional values per serving:

Calories – 229, Fat – 18.8 g, Carbohydrates – 2.9 g, Protein – 13.1 g

Ingredients:

- 16 ounces cauliflower
- Pepper to taste
- Salt to taste
- 4 ounces pancetta, diced
- 4 ounces cheddar cheese, shredded, divided
- 4 ounces Monterey Jack cheese, divided
- ¼ cup scallions, chopped
- 2 tablespoons butter
- ¼ teaspoon garlic powder
- 4 ounces smoked gruyere

Method:

1. Steam the cauliflower until it is soft in the steaming equipment you have.
2. Transfer into a food processor along with salt, pepper, garlic powder and butter.
3. Pulse until smooth. Transfer into a bowl.
4. Place a pan over medium high heat. Add pancetta and cook until crisp. Remove with a slotted spoon and place on a plate that is lined with paper towels.
5. Add cauliflower, half of the cheeses, half the scallions and most of the pancetta into a bowl and mix well.
6. Grease a baking dish with a little oil or butter. Spoon the cauliflower mixture into the baking dish.
7. Sprinkle remaining chesses on top.

8. Bake in a preheated oven at 350° F for about 20-25 minutes.
9. Remove from the oven and let it sit for a few minutes.
10. Sprinkle remaining pancetta and scallions on top and serve.

Coconut Tortillas

Serves: 18-20

Nutritional values per serving:

Calories −63, Fat −4 g, Carbohydrates −6 g, Protein −5 g

Ingredients:

- 1 cup coconut flour
- 2 ½ cups almond milk, unsweetened
- 10 large eggs
- 1 teaspoon sea salt
- Cooking spray

Method:

1. Add all the ingredients into a bowl. Whisk well. Set aside for 5 minutes. The batter should pour easily and should be runny. Add more milk or eggs in equal quantities if required.
2. Place a small skillet or pan over medium heat. Spray with cooking spray. Pour ¼ cup of the prepared batter on the skillet. Swirl the pan so that the batter spreads evenly.
3. Cover the pan with a lid. Cook until the edges begin to get golden brown. Flip sides. Cover and cook until done. Remove and place on a plate.
4. Repeat with the remaining batter to make remaining tortillas.

Creamy Greek Zucchini Patties

Serves: 12

Nutritional values per serving: 1 patty

Calories – 53, Fat – 5 g, Carbohydrates – 2 g, Protein – 2 g

Ingredients:

- 1 pound zucchini, grated
- 1 large handful fresh herbs (mixture of mint, parsley and dill)
- ½ cup feta cheese, crumbled
- ½ teaspoon fine grain sea salt
- 4 teaspoons olive oil, divided
- 1 large egg
- ½ cup almond meal
- ½ teaspoon ground cumin
- Pepper to taste
- Salt to taste

Method:

1. Sprinkle salt over the zucchini and place in a colander. Let it drain for 30-60 minutes.
2. Squeeze the zucchini of excess moisture.
3. Add egg into a large bowl and beat well. Add zucchini, mixed herbs, feta cheese, almond meal, cumin, salt and pepper. Mix well.
4. Place the bowl in the refrigerator for 20-30 minutes.
5. Remove the bowl from the refrigerator. If you find that the mixture is very wet, add a little more of almond meal and mix well.

6. Divide the mixture into 12 equal portions and shape into patties.

7. Place a nonstick pan over medium heat. Add 2 teaspoons oil. When the oil is heated, place a few patties on it. Cook until the underside is golden brown. Flip sides and cook the other side too. Remove with a slotted spoon and place on a plate that is lined with paper towels.

8. Repeat the above step with the remaining patties. Make them in 2-3 batches.

9. Serve.

2-Minute Low Carb English Muffins

Serves: 4

Nutritional values per serving: 1 muffin

Calories –222, Fat –19.4 g, Carbohydrates –4.8 g, Protein –8.3 g

Ingredients:

Wet ingredients:

- 4 tablespoons cashew butter or almond butter or peanut butter
- 2 eggs, beaten
- 2 tablespoons almond milk
- 2 tablespoons butter

Dry ingredients:

- 4 tablespoons almond flour
- 1 teaspoon baking powder
- ¼ teaspoon salt

Method:

1. Add all the dry ingredients into a bowl. Add eggs and milk and whisk until the batter is well combined.
2. Spray 4 ramekins with cooking spray. Set aside.
3. Add almond butter and butter into a microwave safe dish. Microwave on high for 30 seconds or until melted. Mix well. Allow it cool.
4. Add the almond butter mixture into the batter and mix until well combined.
5. Divide the mixture equally and pour into the prepared ramekins.
6. Microwave on high for 2 minutes.

7. When done, let it cool in the ramekins for a few minutes.
8. Serve as it is or toast and serve.

Creamy Ricotta Spaghetti Squash

Serves: 8

Nutritional values per serving: 1-¼ cups

Calories – 129, Fat – 6 g, Carbohydrates – 13 g, Protein – 8 g

Ingredients:

- 2 spaghetti squash, halved, deseeded
- 2 teaspoons garlic powder
- 4 tablespoons fresh basil or parsley, chopped
- 2 cups part skim ricotta cheese
- 2 teaspoons lemon zest, grated
- Salt to taste
- Pepper to taste

Method:

1. Spray the cut part of the spaghetti squash with cooking spray.
2. Place it on a baking sheet with the cut side down.
3. Bake in a preheated oven at 400° F for about 40-50 minutes.
4. When done, using a fork, scrape the squash and add into a bowl.
5. Add ricotta cheese, lemon zest, garlic powder, salt, pepper and basil and mix well.

Spicy Sriracha Roasted Broccoli

Serves: 2

Nutritional values per serving:

Calories – 135, Fat – 12 g, Carbohydrates – 4.5 g, Protein – 2.5 g

Ingredients:

- 2 cups broccoli florets
- 1 teaspoon Sriracha hot sauce
- ½ teaspoon lime juice
- 2 tablespoons Keto friendly mayonnaise
- ½ teaspoon soy sauce or coconut aminos

Method:

1. Steam the broccoli in the steaming equipment you have until it is crisp and bright green in color.
2. Add mayonnaise, soy sauce, hot sauce and lime juice into the baking dish and mix well. Add broccoli and toss well.
3. Broil for 3-4 minutes until slightly brown. Stir and continue broiling for a couple of minutes.
4. Serve hot.

Cheesy Asparagus

Serves: 2

Nutritional values per serving:

Calories – 160, Fat – 12 g, Carbohydrates – 5 g, Protein – 9 g

Ingredients:

- ½ pound asparagus, trimmed
- 2 teaspoons Italian seasoning, divided or to taste
- ¼ cup Parmesan cheese, shredded
- ¼ cup mozzarella cheese, shredded
- 2 teaspoons olive oil
- Sea salt to taste
- Pepper to taste

Method:

1. Place parchment paper or foil on a baking sheet. Spray with a little cooking spray.
2. Place asparagus on the baking sheet. Drizzle oil. Sprinkle 1 teaspoon Italian seasoning, salt and pepper. Toss well.
3. Roast in a preheated oven at 400° F for about 7-9 minutes.
4. Add mozzarella cheese and Parmesan cheese into a bowl and mix. Sprinkle over the asparagus. Sprinkle 1 teaspoon Italian seasoning.
5. Broil for 5-6 minutes or until the cheese melts and is golden brown at spots.

Pork Rind Tortillas

Serves: 6

Nutritional values per serving: 6-inch tortilla

Calories – NA, Fat – 19 g, Carbohydrates – 1 g, Protein – 18 g

Ingredients:

- 2 ounces hot and spicy pork rinds
- 4 eggs
- ½ tablespoons granulated garlic
- 4 ounces cream cheese, softened
- 3 tablespoons water
- ½ tablespoon ground cumin

Method:

1. Add pork rinds into the food processor bowl and process until very fine.
2. Add remaining ingredients and process until a smooth batter is formed.
3. Place a nonstick pan over medium high heat.
4. Spray with cooking spray. When the pan heats, spoon around 1/3 cup of batter on it. Spread out the batter with the back of a spoon or a rubber spatula to around 6 inches diameter or as thin as possible.
5. Cook until golden brown. Once done, flip sides and repeat procedure for the uncooked side.
6. Repeat the above 2 steps with the remaining batter to make 5 more tortillas.
7. You can make the tortillas ahead of time. Wrap it in plastic and freeze until use.

Almond Flour Cream Cheese Crepes

Serves: 4-5

Nutritional values per serving:

Calories – 158, Fat – 13 g, Carbohydrates – 3.04 g, Protein – 6.28 g

Ingredients:

- 2 ounces cream cheese, softened
- 6 tablespoons almond flour
- 2 tablespoons almond milk, unsweetened
- 2 large eggs
- 1 tablespoon swerve sweetener
- Oil or butter to grease the pan
- A pinch salt

Method:

1. Place a sheet of parchment paper on a baking sheet. Set aside.
2. Add almond flour, cream cheese, sweetener, almond milk and salt into a blender. Blend until smooth. Pour into a bowl.
3. Place a nonstick skillet over medium heat. Grease it lightly with butter.
4. When the pan heats, pour 2-3 tablespoons batter and spread with the back of a spoon until it is thin. In a while, when the underside is light brown, loosen the edges with a spatula and carefully lift the crepe and flip sides. Cook the other side until light brown. Remove and place on the prepared baking sheet.
5. Repeat the above step with the remaining batter.

Chapter Eleven: Ketogenic Main Course Recipes

Broccoli Chicken Zucchini Boats

Serves: 4

Nutritional values per serving:

Calories – 476.5, Fat – 34 g, Carbohydrates – 8 g, Protein – 30 g

Ingredients:

- 4 large zucchinis, halved lengthwise
- 6 ounces cheddar cheese, shredded
- 12 ounces rotisserie chicken, shredded
- 2 green onions, thinly sliced
- 8 tablespoons butter, melted
- 2 cups broccoli
- 4 tablespoons sour cream + extra to serve
- Pepper to taste
- Salt to taste

Method:

1. With a spoon, scoop out as much flesh of the zucchini as possible leaving the cases with little flesh (½ -1 cm thick). Repeat with all the zucchini halves.
2. Drizzle about a tablespoon of butter into each zucchini half. Sprinkle salt and pepper.
3. Bake in a preheated oven at 400° F for about 20 minutes.
4. Add chicken, broccoli, salt, pepper and sour cream into a bowl and mix well.

5. When the zucchini is baked, remove from the oven and fill the boats with the chicken filling.
6. Sprinkle cheese over it. Bake for 10-15 minutes or until the cheese melts and is light brown in color.
7. Garnish with green onions and serve with sour cream.

Sesame Ginger Chicken

Serves: 3

Nutritional values per serving:

Calories – 286, Fat – 21 g, Carbohydrates – 3 g, Protein – 19 g

Ingredients:

- ¾ pound chicken thighs, skinless, boneless, chopped into chunks
- ½ tablespoon sesame oil
- ½ tablespoon garlic, minced
- ½ tablespoon rice vinegar
- 1 tablespoon coconut aminos or soy sauce
- ½ tablespoon ginger, minced
- 1 packet Stevia

Method:

1. Add all the ingredients into a Dutch oven. Place the Dutch oven over medium heat.
2. Cook for 15-20 minutes until the chicken is tender.
3. When done, remove chicken with a slotted spoon and place on your cutting board. When cool enough to handle, shred with a pair of forks.
4. Add it back into the pot. Heat thoroughly.
5. Serve as it is or over zucchini noodles or a low carb salad.

Baked Mediterranean Chicken

Serves: 4

Nutritional values per serving:

Calories – 265, Fat – 14.11 g, Carbohydrates – 1.66 g, Protein – 30.87 g

Ingredients:

- 2 medium chicken breasts, halved
- 1 ½ cups baby spinach, chopped
- ½ cup roasted red pepper
- 1 ½ tablespoon butter
- 6 tablespoons light cream cheese
- 1 ½ tablespoon low fat Parmesan cheese, shredded
- Salt to taste
- Pepper powder to taste
- Any herbs and spices of your choice

Method:

1. Pound the chicken breasts pieces with a meat mallet to make cutlets.
2. Add cream cheese, Parmesan, and red pepper into a bowl and mix well.
3. Heat butter in a nonstick skillet. Add spinach. Sauté for a few minutes until the spinach wilts. Remove and add the spinach to the cheese mixture.
4. Add salt, pepper, and herbs. Mix well.
5. Slather a large spoonful of the mixture over each of the chicken cutlets.
6. Roll the cutlets tightly and place with its seam side down on a greased pan.
7. Sprinkle salt and pepper over it.

8. Bake in a preheated oven at 400° F for about 45-60 minutes.
9. Remove from the oven. Serve after 10 minutes.

Bacon, Avocado, and Chicken Sandwich

Serves: 4

Nutritional values per serving:

Calories – 361, Fat – 28.3 g, Carbohydrates – 4 g, Protein – 22 g

Ingredients:

For keto cloud bread:

- 6 large eggs
- ¼ teaspoon cream of tartar
- 1 teaspoon garlic powder
- 6 ounces cream cheese
- ½ teaspoon salt

For the filling:

- 2 tablespoons mayonnaise
- 4 slices bacon
- 4 slices pepper Jack cheese
- ½ medium avocado, peeled, pitted, mashed
- 2 teaspoons Sriracha sauce
- 6 ounces chicken
- 4 grape tomatoes

Method:

1. To make cloud bread: Add the whites and yolks of the eggs in 2 separate bowls.
2. Add salt and cream of tartar to the bowl of whites and whisk until soft peaks are formed.
3. Add cream cheese to the bowl of yolks and whisk until well combined and pale yellow in color.
4. Add the whites into the yolks, a little at a time and fold each time gently.

5. Line a baking sheet with parchment paper. Drop about ¼ cup of the egg mixture on to the baking sheet and shape into squares. Leave a gap between 2 squares. Sprinkle garlic over it.

6. Bake in a preheated oven at 300° F for about 25 minutes.

7. To make filling: Place a skillet over medium heat. Add bacon, salt, pepper and chicken and cook until tender.

8. To assemble: Place the filling over the cloud bread. Spoon some mayonnaise and Sriracha sauce over it. Layer with cheese, tomatoes and finally avocado.

9. Serve immediately.

Zucchini Pizza Casserole

Serves: 4

Nutritional values per serving:

Calories – 211, Fat – 9.1 g, Carbohydrates – 6.4 g, Protein – 26.4 g

Ingredients:

- 1 medium zucchini, shredded
- ¼ cup Parmesan cheese, grated
- 0.65 pound extra lean ground turkey
- ½ tablespoon dried minced onion
- ¼ teaspoon garlic powder
- 10 slices pepperoni
- 1 egg white
- ¾ cup part skim mozzarella cheese, divided
- ½ cup marinara sauce
- ¼ teaspoon Italian seasoning
- Salt to taste

Method:

1. Place zucchini in a colander. Sprinkle salt over it. Mix well. Let the water drain.
2. Squeeze the zucchini of excess moisture.
3. Add zucchini, white, garlic powder, Parmesan cheese, half the mozzarella cheese and Italian seasoning into a bowl and mix well.
4. Transfer into a greased baking dish. Spread the mixture evenly and press it into the dish.
5. Bake in a preheated oven at 400° F for about 20 minutes.
6. Meanwhile, place a skillet over medium heat. Add turkey and dried minced onion and cook until brown.

7. Add marinara sauce and mix well. Transfer into the baking dish over the zucchini layer.
8. Top with remaining cheese. Place pepperoni slices over the cheese. Bake for another 12-15 minutes.

Spinach and Feta Turkey Burgers

Serves: 4

Nutritional values per serving: Without serving options

Calories – 256.2, Fat – 14.6 g, Carbohydrates – 1.4 g, Protein – 28 g

Ingredients:

- 1 large egg
- 1 ounce feta cheese
- 20 ounces ground turkey
- ¼ teaspoon garlic paste
- 2.5 ounces frozen chopped spinach
- Salt to taste
- Pepper to taste

Method:

1. Add all the ingredients into a bowl. Mix well.
2. Divide the mixture into 4 equal portions and shape into patties.
3. Cook on a preheated grill until it is not pink any more in the center of the burger. Cook on both the sides.
4. Serve with keto bun and toppings of your choice.

Mediterranean Pork Chops

Serves: 2

Nutritional values per serving: 2 chops

Calories – 230, Fat – 9 g, Carbohydrates – 9 g, Protein – 28 g

Ingredients:

- 4 thin sliced center cut boneless pork chops
- ½ teaspoon low sodium chicken seasoning
- 3 ounces zucchini, trim the ends
- 3 ounces yellow squash, trim the ends
- ½ cup grape tomatoes, halved
- ½ tablespoon extra-virgin olive oil
- Kosher salt to taste
- Coarsely ground black pepper
- ¼ teaspoon dried oregano
- 2 cloves garlic, thinly sliced
- 2 tablespoons Kalamata olives, pitted, sliced
- 2 tablespoons feta cheese, crumbled
- 2 teaspoons lemon juice
- ½ teaspoon lemon zest, grated
- Cooking spray

Method:

1. Make noodles of the zucchini and yellow squash using a spiralizer or a julienne peeler.
2. Place the tomatoes in a bowl. Add 1-teaspoon olive oil, oregano, salt and pepper to taste. Toss well.
3. Arrange the tomatoes, with the cut side up, on a baking sheet that is lightly greased with cooking spray.
4. Roast in a preheated oven at 300° F for 10 minutes.
5. Add garlic and roast for 4-5 minutes.
6. Transfer into an ovenproof bowl.

7. Place a nonstick skillet over medium high heat. Add the remaining oil. When oil is heated, add zucchini, squash, and salt and sauté until tender. Transfer into the bowl of tomatoes.
8. Lower the temperature of the oven to at 200° F and place the bowl in the oven to keep warm.
9. Place a nonstick skillet over medium high heat. Spray with cooking spray. Cook the pork chops for 1 ½ -2 minutes on each side. Do not cook for longer than this.
10. Place the pork chops on a serving platter.
11. Remove the bowl from the oven. Add olives, lemon juice, and zest. Toss well. Spread the vegetables over the pork chops. Sprinkle feta cheese and serve hot.

Broccoli Rabe & Italian Sausage

Serves: 4

Nutritional values per serving: 2 cups

Calories – 361, Fat – 29 g, Carbohydrates – 3 g, Protein – 20 g

Ingredients:

- 16 ounces Italian sausage
- 4 cloves garlic, thinly sliced
- 4 tablespoons Parmesan cheese, grated
- 2 tablespoons olive oil
- 8 cups raw broccoli rabe, chopped
- Salt to taste
- Pepper to taste

Method:

1. Place a pot of water with a teaspoon of salt over medium heat. Bring to the boil.
2. Add broccoli rabe and cook for a couple of minutes until it gets bright green in color.
3. Drain in a colander.
4. Place a large skillet over medium heat. Add sausage and cook until done.
5. Add oil and garlic and sauté until fragrant.
6. Stir in the drained broccoli rabe and sauté for 2-3 minutes. Turn off the heat.
7. Sprinkle salt and pepper. Sprinkle Parmesan cheese on top and serve right away.

Southwestern Pork Stew

Serves: 2

Nutritional values per serving:

Calories – 386, Fat – 29.5 g, Carbohydrates – 9.7 g, Protein – 19.9 g

Ingredients:

- ½ pound pork shoulder, cooked, sliced
- ½ teaspoon garlic, minced
- 1 teaspoon ground cumin
- 1 teaspoon chili powder
- ½ teaspoon paprika
- Pepper to taste
- Salt to taste
- ½ teaspoon oregano
- 1 bay leaf
- ¼ teaspoon ground cinnamon
- 1 small jalapeño, sliced
- 3 ounces button mushrooms
- ¼ red bell pepper, sliced
- ¼ green bell pepper, sliced
- 1 small onion, sliced
- Juice of a lime
- 1 cup gelatinous bone broth
- ¼ cup strong coffee
- 1 cup chicken broth
- 2 tablespoons tomato paste
- 1 teaspoon olive oil

Method:

1. Place a skillet over high heat. Add oil. When the oil is heated, add onion, garlic, bell peppers, and mushroom and sauté for 4-5 minutes.
2. Add rest of the ingredients and mix well.
3. Lower heat and cover with a lid. Simmer for 15-20 minutes. Stir occasionally.
4. Taste and adjust the seasoning if necessary.
5. Ladle into bowls and serve.

Cheese Pizza Rolls

Serves: 3

Nutritional values per serving:

Calories – 117, Fat – 8 g, Carbohydrates – 3 g, Protein – 11 g

Ingredients:

- 1 cup mozzarella cheese, grated
- 1 tablespoon red bell pepper, chopped
- 1 tablespoon green pepper, chopped
- ¼ cup sausage, cooked, crumbled
- 2 tablespoons keto friendly pizza sauce or marinara sauce
- ½ teaspoon pizza seasoning
- 1 tablespoon white onions, chopped
- 1 grape tomato, sliced

Method:

1. Place parchment paper over a small baking dish. Leave some extra paper on the sides so that it can be easily lifted.
2. Grease the parchment paper with a little oil.
3. Spread cheese all over the baking sheets in a single layer, without any gaps. Sprinkle some pizza seasoning on it.
4. Bake in a preheated oven at 400°F for 15-20 minutes until the cheese browns.
5. Remove the baking dish from the oven and gently try to loosen the pizza crust with the help of a silicone spatula. Begin from the edges and pass it through the middle and entire crust. In case the spatula is not passing

through and the crust not coming off, then place it back in the oven and bake for another 3-5 minutes.

6. Remove the baking dish from the oven.
7. Mix together rest of the ingredients except pizza sauce in a bowl. Spread it over the cheese crust in a thin layer. Pour pizza sauce over it. Sprinkle some pizza seasoning on it.
8. Place it back in the oven and bake for 8-10 minutes.
9. Slice into 3 slices horizontally. Roll each slice with the help of parchment paper. Insert a toothpick in it.
10. Serve.

Low Carb Beef Burritos

Serves: 3

Nutritional values per serving: Without serving options

Calories – 235, Fat – 14 g, Carbohydrates – 4.3 g, Protein – 22 g

Ingredients:

- ½ pound ground beef
- 7 ounces canned or fresh chopped tomatoes
- 1 small red onion, sliced
- 1 clove garlic, crushed
- ½ teaspoon ground chili
- ½ teaspoon smoked paprika
- ½ tablespoon ground cumin
- ½ tablespoon dried coriander
- ½ teaspoon dried oregano

Method:

1. Place a skillet over medium heat. Add oil. When the oil is heated, add onion and garlic and sauté until onions are translucent.
2. Add all the spices, oregano and tomatoes and mix well.
3. Lower heat and cover with a lid. Simmer for 8-10 minutes.
4. Serve with low carb crepes and avocado salsa.

Mexican Shredded Beef

Serves: 6

Nutritional values per serving: Without serving option

Calories – 416, Fat – 27.82 g, Carbohydrates – 1.9 g, Protein – 29.51 g

Ingredients:

- 2 – 2 ½ pounds chuck roast
- 2 tablespoons bacon fat or lard
- ½ cup water
- 2 cloves garlic, minced
- ½ teaspoon chipotle chili powder or ½ tablespoon chili powder
- Salt to taste
- Pepper to taste
- 7.5 ounces canned diced tomatoes
- 1 tablespoon liquid smoke (optional)
- ½ teaspoon ground cumin

Method:

1. Place the rack in the oven in the position next to the lowest position.
2. Sprinkle salt and pepper generously over the roast.
3. Place a Dutch oven over medium heat. Add bacon fat. When it melts, place the roast and cook until brown on all the sides.
4. Add rest of the ingredients and stir. Bring to the boil.
5. Lower heat and simmer until the roast is tender. It will take 3-4 hours. You can also place it in a crockpot and cook.

6. When done, remove the roast and place on your cutting board. When cool enough to handle, shred with a pair of forks. Add the meat into the pot and heat thoroughly.
7. Serve hot over cauliflower rice.

Steak with Mushroom Port Sauce

Serves: 4

Nutritional values per serving: 1 large serving

Calories – 984, Fat – 62 g, Carbohydrates – 6 g, Protein – 102 g

Ingredients:

- 4 pounds Rib eye steak
- 4 ounces heavy cream
- 2 tablespoons butter
- 20 ounces mushrooms
- 8 ounces port wine
- Salt to taste
- Pepper to taste

Method:

1. Season the steak with salt and pepper.
2. Place a large cast iron skillet over high heat. Add butter. When butter melts, place steak and cook for 2 minutes on each side.
3. Place the skillet into a preheated oven.
4. Bake at 450°F for 15-20 minutes or until the internal temperature of the meat shows 135°F when checked with a cooking thermometer. Flip sides half way through baking.
5. Remove the skillet from the oven. Remove the steak, cover with foil and set aside for a while.
6. Pour port wine into the skillet. Scrape the bottom of the skillet to remove any browned bits.
7. Place the skillet over medium heat. Add mushrooms and cream and bring to the boil. Simmer until mushrooms are tender.

8. Spoon the sauce over steak and serve.

Italian Casserole

Serves: 4

Nutritional values per serving:

Calories – 463, Fat – 38 g, Carbohydrates – 5 g, Protein – 24 g

Ingredients:

- ½ pound ground beef
- ¼ pound Italian sausage
- 1 clove garlic, minced
- ¼ pound fresh mushrooms, sliced
- ¼ cup onions, chopped
- Italian seasoning to taste
- ¼ cup mozzarella cheese, shredded
- 4 ounces canned tomato sauce
- Salt to taste
- Pepper powder to taste

For the topping:

- ¼ cup sour cream
- ¼ teaspoon garlic powder
- ¼ cup Parmesan, shredded
- ¼ cup keto friendly mayonnaise
- ¼ teaspoon pepper powder
- ½ cup mozzarella cheese

Method:

1. Grease a baking dish with a little oil. Set aside.
2. Place a nonstick skillet over medium heat. Add the beef, sausage, onions and mushrooms. Sauté until the beef is browned.
3. Add salt and pepper. Mix well. Discard the excess fat from the skillet.

4. Add garlic, tomato sauce, and Italian seasoning into the skillet. Taste and adjust seasoning if necessary.
5. Transfer the contents into the prepared baking dish.
6. Mix together all the ingredients of the topping. Spread over the meat in the baking dish.
7. Bake in a preheated oven at 350° F for 20-30 minutes or until the top is browned.
8. Let it sit in the oven for 10 minutes.
9. Serve.

Easy 30 Minute Keto Chili

Serves: 3

Nutritional values per serving:

Calories – 418, Fat – 28.3 g, Carbohydrates – 5 g, Protein – 32.2 g

Ingredients:

- 1 pound ground beef
- ½ cup tomato sauce
- 1 small onion, diced
- 1 medium green bell pepper
- 4 cups spinach (4 ounces)
- ½ tablespoon olive oil
- ¾ teaspoon chili powder
- ½ teaspoon garlic powder
- ½ tablespoon ground cumin
- 1 teaspoon cayenne pepper
- Pepper to taste
- Salt to taste

Method:

1. Place a skillet over medium heat. Add onion and bell pepper and sauté for about 2 minutes.
2. Add beef, salt and pepper and cook until brown. Add chili powder, garlic powder, cumin and cayenne pepper and sauté for a few seconds until fragrant.
3. Add spinach and cook until it wilts.
4. Add tomato sauce and mix well.
5. Lower heat and simmer for 5-6 minutes. Add Parmesan cheese and stir.
6. Cook for a couple of minutes. Taste and adjust the seasonings if necessary.

7. Serve hot.

Easy Pan Seared Lamb Chops with Mustard Cream Sauce

Serves: 2

Nutritional values per serving:

Calories – 426, Fat – 30 g, Carbohydrates – 4 g, Protein – 31 g

Ingredients:

For pan seared lamb chops:

- ¾ pound lamb chops, trimmed of fat
- ½ tablespoon rosemary, minced
- Salt to taste
- Pepper to taste
- 1 clove garlic, minced
- 1 tablespoon olive oil
- Salt to taste
- Pepper to taste

For mustard cream pan sauce:

- 2 teaspoons minced shallots
- 1 tablespoon brandy
- ½ tablespoon grainy mustard
- 1 teaspoon Worcestershire sauce
- 1 sprig rosemary
- 1 sprig thyme
- Salt to taste
- Pepper to taste
- ¼ cup unsalted beef broth
- 1/3 cup heavy cream
- 1 teaspoon lemon juice
- ½ teaspoon stevia
- 1 tablespoon butter

Method:

1. To make lamb chops: Add rosemary, ½ tablespoon oil and garlic into a bowl and stir.
2. Lay the lamb chops in a baking dish. Sprinkle salt and pepper on it. Place it in a single layer.
3. Spread the garlic rosemary mixture on the lamb chops. Cover the dish with cling wrap and place in the refrigerator for 7-8 hours.
4. Remove from the refrigerator 30 minutes before searing.
5. Place a nonstick pan over medium high heat. Add ½ tablespoon oil. When the oil is heated, add lamb chops in a single layer. Cook in batches if required.
6. Lower the heat to medium and cook for 6-7 minutes on each side or the way you like the chops to be cooked.
7. Remove the lamb chops with a slotted spoon and place on a plate that is lined with paper towels.
8. To make mustard cream pan sauce: Lower the heat to medium low. Add shallots and sauté until translucent.
9. Add broth and brandy and raise the heat to medium heat. When it begins to boil, add mustard, stevia and Worcestershire sauce and mix well.
10. Add rest of the ingredients of the sauce and stir. Simmer until the sauce thickens.
11. Discard the thyme and rosemary sprig.
12. Pour sauce over the chops and serve.

Spicy Tuna Poke Bowl

Serves: 2

Nutritional values per serving:

Calories −340, Fat − 23 g, Net Carbohydrates − 1 g, Protein − 27 g

Ingredients:

- ½ pound fresh ahi tuna, cut into small cubes
- 1 small avocado, peeled, pitted, cubed
- ½ bag miracle noodle rice
- ½ tablespoon sesame oil
- 1 tablespoon soy sauce
- ½ jalapeños (optional), finely chopped
- ¼ cup edamame, shelled
- ½ bunch scallion, finely chopped
- ½ tablespoon black sesame seeds
- ½ tablespoon white sesame seeds
- Salt to taste
- Pepper to taste

For Saravo sauce:

- 1 ½ tablespoons mayonnaise
- 1-2 teaspoons lime juice
- ½ teaspoon Sriracha sauce

Method:

1. Add soy sauce and sesame oil in a bowl and whisk well. Add tuna and toss well. Refrigerate for an hour.
2. Rinse the miracle noodle rice for 10-15 seconds.
3. Place a small saucepan with water over medium heat. Bring to the boil. Add miracle rice and boil for 2 minutes. Drain and transfer rice into a pan.

4. Place the pan over medium heat. Cook until dry.
5. Add avocado into a bowl. Add edamame, scallion, jalapeño, tuna and miracle noodle rice and toss well.
6. To make Saravo sauce: Add mayonnaise, lime juice and Sriracha sauce into a bowl and mix well. Add sauce into the bowl of tuna and fold gently.
7. Divide into bowls. Sprinkle both the sesame seeds over it and serve.

Walnut Crusted Salmon

Serves: 4

Nutritional values per serving:

Calories – 373, Fat – 43 g, Carbohydrates – 4 g, Protein – 20 g

Ingredients:

- 1 cup walnuts
- 2 tablespoons Dijon mustard
- 4 salmon fillets (3 ounces each)
- Salt to taste
- Pepper to taste
- 4 tablespoons sugar free maple syrup
- ½ teaspoon dried dill
- 2 tablespoons olive oil

Method:

1. Place walnuts, mustard and maple syrup in the food processor bowl. Process until a paste is formed. Transfer into a bowl and set aside.
2. Place a skillet over medium heat. Add oil. When the oil is heated, place salmon in the pan with its skin side facing down. Cook for 2 ½ -3 minutes. As it is cooking, spread some walnut mixture to the top part of the fillet.
3. Gently lift the salmon and place in the oven.
4. Bake in a preheated oven at 350° F for 20-30 minutes or until the top is crisp.

Thai Shrimp Curry

Serves: 4

Nutritional values per serving:

Calories – 455, Fat – 31.5 g, Carbohydrates – 13.7 g, Protein – 27 g

Ingredients:

- 4 tablespoons green curry paste
- 2 cups coconut milk
- 10 ounces broccoli florets
- 2 spring onions
- 2 teaspoons ginger, minced
- 2 teaspoons garlic, crushed, roasted
- 1/3 cup fresh cilantro, chopped
- ¼ cup coconut oil
- 2 tablespoons soy sauce
- 2 teaspoons fish sauce
- 2 tablespoons peanut butter
- 2 cups vegetable stock
- 12 ounces precooked shrimp
- Juice of a lemon
- ½ teaspoon xanthan gum
- 1 teaspoon turmeric powder
- 1 cup sour cream to serve

Method:

1. Place a large pan over medium heat. Add oil. When the oil is heated, add ginger and garlic and sauté for a few seconds until fragrant.
2. Add spring onion and sauté for a couple of minutes.
3. Stir in the green curry paste, soy sauce, fish sauce, turmeric powder and peanut butter.

4. Sauté for a couple of minutes. Add xanthan gum, broth and coconut milk. Mix well.
5. Lower heat and simmer for 8-10 minutes or until the gravy thickens.
6. Add broccoli and cook for 5-6 minutes until it is tender. Add and cilantro and cook for 5 minutes.
7. Serve over cauliflower rice, topped with sour cream.

Spicy Shrimp and Cabbage Stir Fry

Serves: 8

Nutritional values per serving: 1/8

Calories – 174, Fat – 3 g, Carbohydrates – 10.2 g, Protein – 25.7 g

Ingredients:

- 2 pounds large or jumbo shrimp, raw, deveined
- 4 tablespoons coconut aminos or soy sauce
- 2 tablespoons rice vinegar
- ½ teaspoon garlic powder
- 1 tablespoons Sriracha sauce or to taste
- 1 teaspoon ground ginger
- 2 teaspoons sesame oil
- A handful fresh cilantro, chopped, to garnish
- 1 head cabbage, shredded
- 2 tablespoons hoisin sauce
- 2 teaspoons sesame seeds, toasted, to garnish

Method:

1. Place a wok or large nonstick skillet over medium high heat. Let the wok heat.
2. Add soy sauce, vinegar, ginger powder, garlic powder, hoisin sauce and Sriracha sauce into a bowl and mix well.
3. Add shrimp into a bowl and add 3-4 tablespoons of the sauce mixture into it. Toss well.
4. Add shrimp into the heated wok. Cook for a couple of minutes until the shrimp are cooked and pink in color. Remove the shrimp and place in a bowl. Set aside.

5. Place the skillet back over high heat. Add cabbage and the remaining sauce and sauté until cabbage wilts.
6. Add the cooked shrimp and stir-fry for a couple of minutes until well combined.
7. Sprinkle sesame seeds and cilantro on top and serve.

Mediterranean Cauliflower Pizza

Serves: 2

Nutritional values per serving:

Calories – 200, Fat – 14 g, Carbohydrates – 10 g, Protein – 11 g

Ingredients:

- 1 pound cauliflower, grated to a rice like texture
- 1 lemon, peeled, quartered
- 1 small egg, lightly beaten
- 3 oil packed sun-dried tomatoes, drained, coarsely chopped
- 3 teaspoons extra virgin olive oil
- 3 tablespoons green or black olives, pitted, sliced
- ½ cup part skim mozzarella cheese
- Salt to taste
- Freshly ground black pepper to taste
- 2 tablespoons fresh basil, thinly sliced
- ½ teaspoon dried oregano

Method:

1. Place a sheet of parchment paper in a pizza pan or baking sheet. Set aside.
2. Place a nonstick skillet over medium high heat. Add 2 teaspoons oil. When the oil is heated, add cauliflower and salt and cook until tender. Do not overcook. Remove from heat and add into a bowl. Set aside to cool.
3. Meanwhile, take a sharp knife and peel the skin of the lemon. Also remove the pitch. Discard the seeds and chop the segment. Add the lemon segments into a bowl. Add tomatoes and olives and toss well.

4. Mix egg, cheese and oregano into the cauliflower. Transfer on to the prepared baking sheet and shape into a round pizza. Sprinkle the remaining oil on it.
5. Bake in a preheated oven at 450° F for 8-12 minutes until the pizza is light brown.
6. Spread the lemon-tomato- olive mixture on top and bake for another 10-15 minutes.
7. Sprinkle basil on top.
8. Slice into 2 equal portions.

Tempeh Lettuce Wraps

Serves: 8

Nutrition values per serving:

Calories - 180, Fat - 9.5 g, Carbohydrates - 12 g, Protein - 13 g

Ingredients:

- 2 packages tempeh, crumbled
- 1 onion, chopped
- 1 red bell pepper, chopped
- 2 heads butter leaf lettuce - 8 leaves
- 2 tablespoons olive oil
- 2 tablespoons garlic, chopped
- 2 tablespoons low sodium soy sauce
- 2 teaspoons garlic powder
- 2 teaspoons ginger powder
- 2 teaspoons onion powder
- Salt to taste

Method:

1. Place a large pan over medium heat. Add oil. When oil is heated, add garlic and sauté for a few seconds until fragrant.
2. Add onions, tempeh and bell pepper and sauté until onions are translucent.
3. Add soy sauce, garlic, ginger powder, onion powder and salt and cook for a couple of minutes. Turn off the heat.
4. Spread the lettuce leaves on your counter top. Spread the tempeh mixture over the leaves. Roll and place on a serving platter with its seam side facing down.
5. The tempeh mixture can be prepared ahead of time and refrigerated until use.
6. Warm the mixture and follow step 4.

7. Serve.

Egg Florentine

Serves: 2

Nutritional values per serving: 2 eggs and 5 tablespoons sauce and without serving option

Calories – 529, Fat – 49 g, Carbohydrates – 3 g, Protein – 20 g

Ingredients:

- 4 large eggs
- 1 cup baby spinach, thinly sliced
- 2 tablespoons extra virgin olive oil
- 2 tablespoons Parmigiano Reggiano cheese, divided
- ¼ teaspoon red pepper flakes or to taste
- 10 tablespoons keto friendly egg fast Alfredo sauce

Method:

1. Place the oven rack in the top part of the oven so that it is closer to the heating element.
2. Place a nonstick skillet over medium high heat. Add oil. When the oil is heated, add eggs and cook the eggs sunny side up.
3. Take 2 small baking dishes. Grease the dishes with oil. Pour ¼ the egg fast Alfredo sauce in each of the dishes. Gently slide 2 eggs in each dish.
4. Pour remaining Alfredo sauce on the eggs. Sprinkle 1-tablespoon cheese in both the dishes.
5. Place in a preheated oven and broil for 2-3 minutes.
6. Remove from the oven and sprinkle spinach on top. Sprinkle some more cheese if desired and red pepper flakes.
7. Serve with keto bread.

Grain Free Mac and Cheese

Serves: 6

Nutritional values per serving:

Calories – 627, Fat – 52 g, Carbohydrates – 14 g, Protein – 25 g

Ingredients:

- ¾ cup crème fraiche
- 3 tablespoons yellow mustard
- Pepper to taste
- Salt to taste
- 1 ½ pounds jicama, cut into ¼ inch cubes
- 4 ½ cups Sharp cheddar cheese, shredded
- ¾ cup heavy cream
- ¾ cup onion, minced

Method:

1. Add crème fraiche, salt, pepper, cream and mustard into a bowl and mix well.
2. Add onion and jicama and mix well. Add cheese and mix until well combined.
3. Transfer into a baking dish.
4. Bake in a preheated oven at 350° F for 40-50 minutes.

Chapter Twelve: Ketogenic Dessert Recipes

Strawberry Ice Cream with Chocolate Sauce

Serves: 4

Nutritional values per serving: For ice cream

Calories - 213, Fat – 17.4 g, Carbohydrates – 15.8 g, Protein – 4 g

Nutritional values per serving: For chocolate sauce

Calories - 58, Fat – 6.1 g, Carbohydrates – 1.8 g, Protein – 0.7 g

Ingredients:

For ice cream:

- 2 cans (16 ounces each) light coconut milk
- 1 teaspoon pure vanilla extract
- 2 cups strawberries
- White stevia to taste

For chocolate sauce:

- 4 tablespoons coconut cream
- 2 teaspoons coconut oil
- 4 teaspoons cacao powder
- White stevia to taste

Method:

1. To make ice cream: Add all the ingredients of ice cream into the blender and blend until smooth.
2. Pour into an ice cream maker and follow the manufacturer's instructions and churn the ice cream. It will be of soft serve consistency. Alternately, pour into a freezer safe bowl. Cover with a lid and freeze until it is of soft serve consistency.
3. To make chocolate sauce: Add all the ingredients of chocolate sauce into a bowl and mix well.
4. Divide ice cream into 4 bowls. Divide and pour the sauce over the ice cream and serve.

Raspberry Cheesecake Bites Coated in Chocolate

Serves: 8

Nutritional values per serving:

Calories - 134, Fat – 12.8 g, Carbohydrates – 3.1 g, Protein – 2.5 g

Ingredients:

- 4.4 ounces mascarpone cheese or full fat cream cheese or creamed coconut milk
- ½ teaspoon vanilla extract or ¼ teaspoon vanilla bean powder
- ¼ cup almond flour
- 10 drops stevia (optional)
- ½ cup frozen raspberries
- 1 tablespoons stevia or swerve, powdered
- 2 tablespoons coconut flour

For coating:

- 0.7 ounce cacao butter or extra virgin coconut oil
- 1.4 ounces 90% dark chocolate

Method:

1. Add mascarpone cheese, raspberries and stevia into the food processor bowl. Process until smooth.
2. Add almond flour and coconut flour and process until well combined.
3. Spoon into ice tray (about 2 tablespoons in each ice mold). Freeze for an hour.

4. For coating: Add coconut oil and dark chocolate into a heatproof bowl. Place the bowl in a double boiler. Stir occasionally until the mixture melted.
5. Remove the bowl from the double boiler.
6. Line a tray with parchment paper.
7. Remove the cheesecake from the ice tray and dip into the chocolate mixture.
8. Place on the prepared tray. Freeze until set. Transfer into an airtight container.
9. Store in the freezer until use.

Maple Pecan Muffins

Serves: 22

Nutritional values per serving:

Calories – 208, Fat – 20.7 g, Carbohydrates – 5.15 g, Protein – 4.8 g

Ingredients:

- 2 cups almond flour
- 1 ½ cups pecan halves
- 4 large eggs
- 4 teaspoons maple extract
- 1 teaspoon baking soda
- ½ teaspoon liquid stevia
- 1 cup golden flaxseed
- 1 cup coconut oil
- ½ cup stevia
- 2 teaspoons vanilla extract
- 1 teaspoon apple cider vinegar

Method:

1. Add pecans into the food processor bowl. Pulse until it is chopped into small pieces. Set aside 1/3 of the nuts and add the rest into a mixing bowl.
2. Add almond flour, baking soda and flaxseed into the bowl of pecans.
3. Mix together rest of ingredients in another bowl. Pour into the bowl of almond flour mixture and whisk until well combined.
4. Line 22 muffin molds with cupcake liners. Divide the batter among the molds.
5. Sprinkle the pecans that were set aside.
6. Bake in a preheated oven at 325° F for about 20- 25 minutes.

7. Remove from the oven.
8. Loosen the edges of the muffin with a knife. Invert on to a plate.
9. Cool and serve.

Dark Chocolate Fat Bombs

Serves: 34

Nutritional values per serving:

Calories – 104.7, Fat – 11.9 g, Carbohydrates – 0.4 g, Protein – 0.2 g

Ingredients:

- 1 cup coconut oil
- 4 tablespoons Hershey's cocoa special dark
- Stevia extract to taste
- 1 cup unsalted butter
- 1 teaspoon vanilla extract

Method:

1. Add butter and oil to a microwave safe bowl. Microwave for 30-40 seconds until the mixture melts.
2. Stir well. Add cocoa, vanilla and stevia extract and stir until well combined.
3. Pour into 34 small silicone molds or silicone tray. Freeze for a couple of hours until it is set.
4. If you pour in the tray, then chop into 34 equal pieces.
5. Remove from the mold and transfer into an airtight container. Freeze until use.

Coconut Mocha Mug Cake

Serves: 2

Nutritional values per serving:

Calories – 418, Fat – 40 g, Carbohydrates – 11 g, Protein – 10 g

Ingredients:

- 2 large eggs, at room temperature
- 4 tablespoons almond flour
- 14 drops stevia
- 4 tablespoons butter, at room temperature
- 2 tablespoons stevia
- 1 teaspoon baking powder
- 2 tablespoons cocoa powder, unsweetened
- 4 teaspoons coconut flour
- 2 tablespoons unsweetened shredded coconut + extra to serve
- 1 teaspoon instant coffee
- 2 tablespoons coconut milk, at room temperature

Method:

1. Add all the ingredients into a bowl and mix well.
2. Divide equally and pour into 2 mugs.
3. Microwave on high for 70 seconds.
4. Cool for a while. Run a knife around the edges of the mug. Invert on to a plate.
5. Garnish with shredded coconut and serve.

Blackberry Pudding

Serves: 4

Nutritional values per serving:

Calories – 477.5, Fat – 43.5 g, Carbohydrates – 10.66 g,
Protein – 9 g

Ingredients:

Dry ingredients:

- ½ cup coconut flour
- ½ teaspoon baking powder

Wet ingredients:

- 10 large egg yolks
- 4 tablespoons butter
- 4 teaspoons lemon juice
- ½ cup blackberries
- 20 drops liquid stevia
- 4 tablespoons coconut oil
- 4 tablespoons heavy cream
- Zest of 2 lemons, grated
- 4 tablespoons stevia

Method:

1. Mix together all the dry ingredients into a bowl and set aside.
2. Add butter and coconut oil into a bowl and mix well. Set aside.
3. Add yolks into a bowl and beat until they turn pale yellow in color. Add stevia and stevia and beat until it is dissolved.

4. Add cream, lemon juice and lemon zest into the coconut oil butter mixture. Beat until well combined. Add the egg yolk mixture and beat again.
5. Add the dry ingredients into the above mixture and mix until well combined.
6. Grease 4 ramekins and pour the batter among the ramekins. Place blackberries on top. Push it lightly into the batter.
7. Bake in a preheated oven at 350° F for about 20- 25 minutes.
8. Remove from the oven and cool completely.
9. Run a knife around the edges of the ramekins. Invert on to a plate.
10. Serve.

Strawberry Shortcake

Serves: 10

Nutritional values per serving:

Calories −273.2, Fat −25.96 g, Carbohydrates −4.42 g, Protein −6.64 g

Ingredients:

For keto puff cakes:

- 6 large eggs
- ½ teaspoon baking powder
- 4 tablespoons stevia
- ½ teaspoon vanilla extract
- 6 ounces cream cheese

For filling:

- 2 cups heavy cream, whipped
- 20 strawberries, chopped

Method:

1. Add yolks into a bowl and whites into another bowl.
2. Line a baking sheet with parchment paper and set aside.
3. Beat egg whites with an electric mixer until soft peaks are formed.
4. Add vanilla, cream cheese, stevia and baking powder into the bowl of yolks.
5. Beat again until well combined. Spoon whites into the cream cheese mixture. Fold gently.
6. Spread on the prepared baking sheet.
7. Bake in a preheated oven at 300°F for about 30-35 minutes or until done.

8. Cool for at least an hour before serving.
9. Chop into 20 equal squares.
10. Mix together cream and strawberries.
11. Sandwich the strawberry cream mixture between 2 squares of shortcake and serve.

Dreamsicle Dessert

Serves: 12

Nutritional values per serving:

Calories – 25.7, Fat – 0 g, Carbohydrates – 5.7 g, Protein – 1 g

Ingredients:

- 2 small packages (1.4 ounces each) sugar-free, fat free vanilla pudding mix
- 16 ounces low fat or fat free whipped topping (Cool Whip)
- 2 small packages (0.3 ounces each) sugar free orange Jell-O

Method:

1. Make the orange Jell-O according to the instructions on the package.
2. Add pudding mix powder to the Jell-O. Whisk until smooth. Add the whipped topping and fold gently until the topping is well mixed in the Jell-O but do not beat.
3. Spoon into 12 dessert bowls.
4. Chill for at least 3 hours or until set.
5. Serve.

Chocolate Ice Cream

Serves: 4

Nutritional values per serving:

Calories – 318, Fat – 26.8 g, Carbohydrates – 9.1 g, Protein – 3 g

Ingredients:

- 2 cans coconut milk
- 2 teaspoons chocolate stevia
- 4 tablespoons cocoa powder, unsweetened
- A pinch salt
- Cacao nibs (optional)

Method:

1. Add all the ingredients to a blender. Blend until smooth.
2. Pour into an ice cream maker and churn the ice cream following the manufacturer's instructions. Alternately, pour into a freezer safe container and cover with a lid.
3. Freeze until firm.
4. Remove from the freezer around 30 minutes before serving.
5. Scoop into bowls and serve.

Frost Bite Cookies

Serves: 12

Serves:

Nutritional values per serving:

Calories – 91, Fat – 9.4 g, Carbohydrates – 2 g, Protein – 1.2 g

Ingredients:

- ¼ cup coconut oil or butter
- 1 egg
- 1 teaspoon vanilla
- 14 tablespoons swerve sweetener
- ½ cup cocoa, unsweetened
- 1/8 teaspoon sea salt

For frost bite dip:

- 2 ounces edible cocoa butter
- 1/8 teaspoon almond extract
- ½ teaspoon vanilla extract
- 6 tablespoons swerve confectioners
- 1/8 teaspoon sea salt

Method:

1. Add butter and sweetener into a mixing bowl. Beat until smooth and creamy.
2. Add eggs and beat until well combined. Add cocoa, salt and vanilla extract. Mix well until dough is formed.
3. Divide the mixture into 12 equal portions and shape into balls. Flatten the balls and place on a baking sheet. Leave a gap between the cookies.

4. Bake in a preheated oven at 350° F for about 10 minutes. Remove the baking sheet from the oven and cool completely. Remove the cookies and set aside.
5. To make frost bite dip: Melt the cocoa butter in a double boiler over medium heat. Add rest of the ingredients and mix well. You can also melt in a microwave.
6. Spread the dip over the top part cookies and set aside for a while to set.

Day 1:

Breakfast – Cheese and Ham Waffles

Lunch – Chicken and Kale Soup

Snack – Coconut Milkshake

Dinner – Zucchini Pizza Casserole

Day 2:

Breakfast – Bacon, Cheese and Egg Cups

Lunch – Chicken Salad Picnic Eggs

Snack – Creamy Red Gazpacho

Dinner – Mediterranean Chopped Salad

Day 3:

Breakfast – Apple and Brie Crepes

Lunch – Grilles Vegetable Salad with Olive oil and Feta

Snack – Blackberry Cheesecake Smoothie

Dinner – Broccoli Chicken Zucchini Boats

Day 4:

Breakfast – Zucchini and Chicken quiche

Lunch – Avgolemono

Snack – Maple Pecan Muffins

Dinner – Curried Chicken Salad

Day 5:

Breakfast – Blueberry Coconut Porridge

Lunch – Grain Free Mac and Cheese

Snack – Mini Cheese Balls

Dinner – Lemon Blueberry Chicken Salad

Day 6:

Breakfast – Lemon Poppy Seed Pancakes

Lunch – Cream of Chicken Soup with Bacon

Snack – Low Carb Pizza Bites

Dinner – Egg Florentine

Day 7:

Breakfast – Feta and Pesto Omelet

Lunch – Mock Potato Salad

Snack – Blackberry Pudding

Dinner – Spicy Tuna Poke Bowl

Day 8:

Breakfast – Perfect Scramble

Lunch – Broccoli Cheese Soup

Snack – Spicy Chicken Nuggets

Dinner – Tempeh Lettuce Wraps

Day 9:

Breakfast – Blackberry Egg Bake

Lunch – Curried Chicken Salad

Snack – Strawberry Shortcake

Dinner – Mediterranean Cauliflower Pizza

Day 10:

Breakfast – Creamy Cauliflower and Ground Beef Skillet

Lunch – Mediterranean Cauliflower Pizza

Snack – Italian Style Zucchini Rolls

Dinner – Lemon Blueberry Chicken Salad

Day 11:

Breakfast – Morning Meatloaf

Lunch – Mediterranean Chopped Salad

Snack – Marinated Olives and Feta

Dinner – Thai Shrimp Curry

Day 12:

Breakfast – Breakfast BLT Salad

Lunch – Easy Pan seared Lamb Chops with Mustard Cream Sauce

Snack – Blackberry Pudding

Dinner – Easy 30-minute Keto Chili

Day 13:

Breakfast – Chocolate Waffles

Lunch – Crunchy and Nutty Cauliflower Salad

Snack – Pork Rind Tortillas

Dinner – Tempeh Lettuce Wraps

Day 14:

Breakfast – Liver, Sausage and Eggs

Lunch – Easy 30-minute Keto Chili

Snack – Coconut Mocha Mug Cake

Dinner – Egg Florentine

Day 15:

Breakfast – Coconut Flour Porridge Breakfast Cereal

Lunch – Roasted Bell Pepper and Cauliflower Soup

Snack – Creamy Ricotta Spaghetti Squash

Dinner – Mock Potato Salad

Day 16:

Breakfast – Cheese and Ham Waffles

Lunch – Chicken Cobb Salad

Snack – Pesto Keto Crackers

Dinner – Sesame Ginger Chicken

Day 17:

Breakfast – Bacon, Cheese and Egg Cups

Lunch – Curried Chicken Salad

Snack – Avocado Balls

Dinner – Easy Russian Slaw

Day 18:

Breakfast – Apple and Brie Crepes

Lunch – Zucchini Pizza Casserole

Snack – 2-Minute Low Carb English Muffins

Dinner – Low Carb Beef Burritos

Day 19:

Breakfast – Zucchini and Chicken quiche

Lunch – Walnut Crusted Salmon

Snack – Frost Bite Cookies

Dinner – Mexican Shredded Beef

Day 20:

Breakfast – Blueberry Coconut Porridge

Lunch – Spicy Shrimp and Cabbage Stir Fry

Snack – Healthy Keto Green Smoothie

Dinner – Spinach and Feta Turkey Burgers

Day 21:

Breakfast – Lemon Poppy Seed Pancakes

Lunch – Sesame Ginger Chicken

Snack – Raspberry Cheesecake Bites coated in Chocolate

Dinner – Pork Rind Tortillas

Day 22:

Breakfast – Strawberry and Rhubarb Pie Smoothie

Lunch – Broccoli Rabe and Italian Sausage

Snack – Spicy Sriracha Roasted Broccoli

Dinner – Southwestern Pork Stew

Day 23:

Breakfast – Perfect Scramble

Lunch – Spinach and Feta Turkey Burgers

Snack – Creamy Greek Zucchini Patties

Dinner – Bacon, Avocado, and Chicken Sandwiches

Day 24:

Breakfast – Blackberry Egg Bake

Lunch – Steak with Mushroom Port Sauce

Snack – Cheesy Cauliflower gratin

Dinner – Crunchy and Nutty Cauliflower Salad

Day 25:

Breakfast – Creamy Cauliflower and Ground Beef Skillet

Lunch – Baked Mediterranean Chicken

Snack – Cauliflower, Cheese, and Onion Croquette

Dinner – Walnut Crusted Salmon

Day 26:

Breakfast – Morning Meatloaf

Lunch – Walnut Crusted Salmon (leftover)

Snack – Green Lemon Smoothie

Dinner – Thai Shrimp Curry with Rice

Day 27:

Breakfast – Breakfast BLT Salad

Lunch – Kale and Sausage Soup

Snack – Coconut Tortillas

Dinner – Italian Casserole

Day 28:

Breakfast – Healthy Green Shake

Lunch – Southwestern Pork Stew

Snack – Cheesy Asparagus

Dinner – Zucchini Pizza Casserole

Day 29:

Breakfast – Liver, Sausage and Eggs

Lunch – Zucchini Pizza Casserole (leftover)

Snack – Almond Flour Cream Cheese Crepes

Dinner – Low Carb Burritos

Day 30:

Breakfast – Raspberry Avocado Smoothie

Lunch – Creamy Garlic Chicken Soup

Snack – Colcannon

Dinner – Grilled Vegetable Salad with Olive oil and Feta

Conclusion

That brings us to the end of this book. I am aware that it was a lot of information to process in one go! Don't worry if most of it went over your head. Use this book as your Keto guide and go over each section patiently.

The bottom line is that this diet is capable of improving the quality of your health in no time and you are doing yourself a huge favor by adopting this diet!

I sincerely hope that you found this book useful. I wish you good luck and urge you to be patient and consistent. You will definitely reap the fruits of your efforts.

Thank you again for purchasing this book!

Finally, if you enjoyed this book then I'd like to ask you for a favor. Will you be kind enough to leave a review for this book on Amazon? It would be greatly appreciated!

Here is the link on Amazon:
https://www.amazon.com/dp/1973524112/

Please also see the chapters **Recommended Reading, Recommended Websites, and Recommended Products and Solutions.**

Thank you and good luck!

Recommended Reading

Here are some books that you may find interesting to read:

1. **Reduce Blood Pressure Naturally with The Beginner's Dash Diet:** Includes a Dash Diet Eating Plan Chart, 140 Dash Diet Recipes for Easy Meal Planning, and FAQs
2. The Beginner's Mediterranean Diet for Healthy Weight Loss: 30 Day Guide with 90 Easy to Cook Recipes

Recommended Websites (under development)

Here are some websites that may be of interest to you:

1. https://dogloversforlife.com
2. https://healthylivingforadults.com

Recommended Products and Solutions (Future)

Made in the USA
San Bernardino, CA
18 May 2018